HKP SPORT SCIENCE MONOGRAPH SERIES
Volume 2

Biological Effects of Physical Activity

R. Sanders Williams, MD
Andrew G. Wallace, MD
Duke University Medical Center
Editors

Human Kinetics Books
Champaign, Illinois

Library of Congress Cataloging-in-Publication Data

PepsiCo Foundation Conference on Fitness and Health (1st : 1988 : Duke University)
 Biological effects of physical activity / edited by R. Sanders Williams, Andrew G. Wallace.
  p. cm. — (HKP sport science monograph series, ISSN 0894-4229; v. 2)
 "Proceedings of the First Biennial PepsiCo Foundation Conference on Fitness and Health held at Duke University, May 9th and 10th, 1988, Durham, North Carolina"—T.p. verso.
 Includes bibliographies.
 ISBN 0-87322-218-0
 1. Exercise—Physiological aspects—Congresses. 2. Physical fitness—Congresses. I. Williams, R. Sanders (Robert Sanders), 1948- .
II. Wallace, Andrew G., 1935- . III. Title. IV. Series.
 [DNLM: 1. Exercise—congresses. 2. Physical Fitness—congresses.
WB 541 P424b 1988]
QP301.P374 1988
612'.04—dc19
DNLM/DLC
for Library of Congress   89-1757
                                                                            CIP

Proceedings of the First Biennial PepsiCo Foundation Conference on Fitness and Health, held at Duke University, Durham, North Carolina, May 9–10, 1988.

ISBN: 0-87322-218-0
ISSN: 0894-4229

Copyright © 1989 by Human Kinetics Publishers, Inc.

Production Director: Ernie Noa
Managing Editor: Kathy Kane
Copyeditor: Molly Bentsen
Typesetter: Impressions, Inc.
Text Design: Keith Blomberg

Printed in the United States of America

3 2 1

Human Kinetics Books
A Division of Human Kinetics Publishers, Inc.
Box 5076, Champaign, IL 61825-5076
1-800-DIAL-HKP
1-800-334-3665 (in Illinois)

Contents

HKP Sport Science Monograph Series

Ten years ago I completed a series of studies on competitive anxiety that validated the Sport Competition Anxiety Test (SCAT). I wanted to publish all this work in one place rather than chopping it into shorter research articles that would meet the space restrictions of scholarly journals. Because a place to publish monograph length research did not exist then in the sport sciences, I published it as the third book of the then neophyte Human Kinetics Publishers.

The need for a research monograph series continues today and was brought back to my attention by Professor Robert Malina when he sought to have the cumulative work of the *Physical Growth and Motor Performance of Belgian Boys Followed Longitudinally Between 12 and 18 Years of Age* published in its entirety. The report of that project is the first publication in the new *HKP Sport Science Monograph Series*. The series is an extension of Human Kinetics Publishers' scholarly journal program.

The *HKP Sport Science Monograph Series* is another endeavor to provide a useful communication channel for recording extensive research programs by sport scientists. Many publishers have discontinued publishing monographs because they have proven uneconomical. It is my hope that with the cooperation of authors, the use of electronic support systems, and the purchase of these monographs by sport scientists and libraries we can continue this series over the years.

The series will publish original research reports and reviews of literature that are sufficiently extensive not to lend themselves to reporting in available research journals. Subject matter pertinent both to the broad fields of the sport sciences and to physical education are considered appropriate for the monograph series, especially research in

- Sport biomechanics,
- Sport physiology,
- Motor behavior (including motor control and learning, motor development, and adapted physical activity),
- Sport psychology,
- Sport sociology, and
- Sport pedagogy.

Authors who wish to publish in the monograph series should submit two copies of the complete manuscript to the publisher. All manuscripts must conform to the current *APA Publication Manual* and be of a length between 120 and 300 doublespaced manuscript pages. The manuscript will be sent to two reviewers who will follow a review process similar to that used for scholarly journals. The decision with regard to the manuscript's acceptability will be based on its judged contribution to knowledge and on economic feasibility. Publications that are accepted, after all required revisions are made, must be submitted to the publisher on computer disk for electronic transfer to typesetting. No royalties will be paid for monographs published in this series.

Authors wishing to submit a manuscript to the monograph series or desiring further information should write to: Monograph Editor, Human Kinetics Publishers, Box 5076, Champaign, IL 61825 for further details.

Rainer Martens

Preface

In 1986 the PepsiCo Foundation awarded a major lead grant to Duke University to help establish a Center for Fitness Research. As a part of that grant, PepsiCo endowed a biennial conference to be held at Duke University, Durham, North Carolina. This book contains the Proceedings of the First Biennial PepsiCo Foundation Conference.

The purpose of this conference was to bring together in one setting leading scientists from around the world who are working on the biological and psychological effects of exercise and leaders from the corporate sector who have significant experience in implementing fitness programs and other wellness strategies in the workplace. This mixture of participants is unusual, but was designed to achieve specific objectives. First, we wanted this and subsequent PepsiCo conferences to discuss the biology of exercise and exercise training at the highest scientific level. Second, we wanted to expose corporate leaders to the best scientific thought. Third, we wanted the scientific community to see how the results of its research are being applied and to learn what hurdles need to be overcome to effectively promote the beneficial effects of exercise as a strategy for achieving better health.

Finally, by holding this conference at the Duke University School of Medicine and inviting leaders from other academic health centers, we wanted to stimulate and promote a broader commitment to fitness-related research and education in the medical schools of the United States. Publication of these Proceedings will capture the content of the meeting in a format that will be useful to both the academic and the corporate world.

Donald M. Kendall

R. Sanders Williams, MD

Andrew G. Wallace, MD

Part I

A Scientific Perspective

Oxygen Transport During Exercise:
Role of the Cardiovascular System

Bengt Saltin
University of Copenhagen
Copenhagen, Denmark

A knowledge about the capacity of the various links in the circulatory system in the human or any species would aid in understanding the principles for control of the cardiovascular system when under load, such as during exercise. If the heart of a species has the capacity to supply blood flow and maintain blood pressure when most vascular beds of the body are maximally dilated, then control principles are likely to be different than if the conductance of the periphery vastly surpasses the central circulatory capacity. In humans it has been established that the various links of the circulatory system are closely interrelated; i.e., correlation coefficients are around .9 or above when the amount of hemoglobin, blood volume, heart volume, and stroke volume as well as muscle capillary density and muscle mass are related to each other or to maximal values for cardiac output or oxygen uptake (Holmgren & Åstrand, 1966). The conclusion then is that there is a good balance and match between central and peripheral capacities. During exercise a maximal vasodilation of muscle can thus be allowed.

Indeed, recently it has been proposed that the blood flow to muscles is excessive during maximal whole body exercise. This notion was based on observations of some oxygen remaining in the venous blood returning from contracting muscles during exhaustive exercise at sea level and various altitudes (Wagner, 1988; Wagner et al., 1986).

Also, the opposite view has been voiced; that is, the heart and the cardiac output are insufficient for the huge potential for a flow of the skeletal muscle (Rowell, Saltin, Kiens, & Christensen, 1986). In this article the evidence to support this latter view will be presented. It will be argued that although it is believed that the heart limits oxygen transport in intense whole body exercise of man and thus maximal oxygen uptake, this view may well be compatible with a close statistical coupling between links of the cardiovascular system, as well as with some oxygen remaining

3

in the venous blood that drains contracting skeletal muscle. Further, different options for control of the peripheral resistance during intense exercise with large muscle groups will be discussed, as will some practical consequences related to training the cardiovascular system and endurance.

Pulmonary Function

During muscular exercise (at sea level) an almost complete oxygen saturation of the arterial blood is maintained. This applies for very intense exercise, performed by untrained or very well-trained individuals (Table 1). This high degree of saturation has its price. As the work load is increased, a larger alveolar arterial oxygen gradient is necessary, which is secured through hyperventilation. At rest and during light exercise the relationship between oxygen taken up and ventilation is one L oxygen per 20 L ventilation. This ratio increases at the same time as the pH of the blood starts to decline, and it reaches 30 to 40 L per L O_2 at maximal exercise. The conclusions must be that the pulmonary function is adequate even during very intense physical exercise and that enough oxygen is transferred in the lungs to avoid arterial desaturation, even though the price is a highly increased ventilation.

Though no one has actually questioned this description, new dimensions have been added to it since a report that some runners show a clear arterial desaturation during exercise (Table 2; Dempsey, 1986; Dempsey, Hanson, & Henriksson, 1984). In fact, a few similar observations in well-trained individuals were described in 1964 (Rowell, Taylor, Wang, & Carlson). In these studies the most interesting observation is that the desaturation occurs at a relatively light work load, which is explained by the fact that the well-trained individuals did not show the "normal" hyperventilation. It is noteworthy that when nitrogen is replaced with the lighter gas helium, the runners who earlier showed hypoventilation start to hyperventilate and an increase in the arterial oxygen content is seen (Dempsey et al., 1984).

Runners showing arterial desaturation have less oxygen in their arterial blood. This is compensated for by a somewhat higher cardiac output and a larger muscle blood flow at a given work load (Saltin, Kiens, Savard, & Pedersen, 1986). This means that the work of the heart becomes elevated to compensate for the lower ventilatory performance. As described later, the cardiac output of an individual has an upper limit, which means that the maximal amount of oxygen offered to the tissues by the heart is reduced by the degree of arterial desaturation. In return breathing is less "costly." The exact numbers of this calculation are unknown. However, it is most likely that athletes, and especially endurance athletes who do not maintain their arterial oxygen saturation, are impaired.

The observations by Dempsey and coworkers (Dempsey, 1986; Dempsey et al., 1984) indicate that well-trained individuals operate close to their upper limit of pulmonary oxygen transport. However, it is important to emphasize that arterial desaturation is unusual at sea level. In

Table 1   Some Respiratory and Circulatory Variables Observed in Men in Different Physical Training Conditions

Variable	Control	After bedrest	After training	Olympic athletes
Maximal oxygen uptake (l · min)	3.30	2.43	3.91	5.38
Maximal voluntary ventilation (l · min)	191	201	197	219
Transfer coefficient for O_2 (ml · min)/ (mmHg)	96	83	86	95
Arterial O_2 capacity (vol %)	21.9	20.5	20.8	22.4
Maximal cardiac output (l · min)	20.0	14.8	22.8	30.4
Stroke volume (ml)	104	74	120	167
Maximal heart rate (b · min)	192	197	190	182
Systemic arteriovenous O_2 difference (vol %)	16.2	16.5	17.1	18.0

Note. From "Cardiovascular Adaptations to Physical Training" by C.G. Blomqvist and B. Saltin, 1983, *Annual Review of Physiology,* **45**, pp. 169–189.

Table 2   Summary of Blood Gas Data from Dempsey et al. (1984; 1986) and Ekblom and Hermansen's (1968) Studies of Very Well-Trained Endurance Athletes Performing Short Lasting Exhaustive Exercise

	Exhaustive exercise			
	PaO_2 (mmHg)	SaO_2 (%)	$PaCO_2$ (mmHg)	pH
Dempsey et al. (1984)				
n=4	91	95	29	7.26
n=9 $\dot{V}O_2$max = 71.9	77	84	33	7.29
n=3 (ml · kg^{-1} · min^{-1})	58	76	37	7.31
Ekblom and Hermansen (1968)				
n=8 $\dot{V}O_2$max = 74.6		93		
(ml · kg^{-1} · min^{-1})		(89–94)		

Ekblom and Hermansen's study (1968) of very well-trained skiers and runners, who had higher maximal oxygen uptake than the runners in the study by Dempsey et al., all had an arterial oxygen saturation of 89% or more during maximal exercise (Table 1).

Circulation

The detailed description of the circulatory adaptation to muscular exercise has been studied from the beginning of the century (Armstrong, Delp, Goljan, & Laughlin, 1987). The most important findings are that cardiac output increases linearly with increasing work load (and oxygen uptake) and that the highest attainable values of an individual can be markedly affected by physical training (Table 1). Maximal cardiac output of physically inactive individuals is only 30% to 40% of that of the most well-trained. The size of the stroke volume determines the size of the cardiac output, as the maximal heart rate is the same or slightly lower after training.

In the last 10 to 15 years the focus has been on the question of whether a balance exists between maximal cardiac output and the perfusion capacity of skeletal muscles. The first and more certain evidence for the existence of a discrepancy between the pump capacity of the heart and the muscular conductance came in 1977, when Secher, Clausen, and Klausen published results showing a reduction in leg blood flow when adding arm exercise to leg exercise (Figure 1). This occurred in spite of an unchanged arterial blood pressure and regardless of the fact that the local factors influencing the vasodilation were increased. These data suggest that if the fraction of muscle mass involved in the exercise surpasses a certain critical limit, vasoconstriction is elicited in spite of a large accumulation of vasodilator substances.

In subsequent studies attempts have been made to determine more precisely the maximal perfusion capacity of skeletal muscles. If the pump capacity of the heart is a limiting factor, it will in these experiments be important only to involve a small fraction of the muscle mass in the exercise (Andersen, Adams, Sjøgaard, Thorboe, & Saltin, 1985) and be able to quantitate the muscle mass involved in the exercise. In a study where exercise was performed with the knee extensors of one leg, measurements of blood flow to (a. femoralis) or from (v. femoralis) the muscle showed that during exhaustive exercise blood flow can reach 5 to 6 L · min^{-1} (Andersen & Saltin, 1985; Wesche, 1986). The muscle mass involved in the exercise weighed 2 to 3 kg. The muscle perfusion is then 1.5 to 2 L · kg^{-1} · min^{-1}. Evidently this means that if all the skeletal muscles (30 kg in a man of 70 kg) were to maintain that high a blood flow it would demand a cardiac output of over 45 to 50 L · min^{-1}. A cardiac output of that size has never been demonstrated (Table 1). It can therefore be concluded that there is an imbalance between the pump capacity of the heart and the maximal conductance of the muscles. The latter is markedly higher.

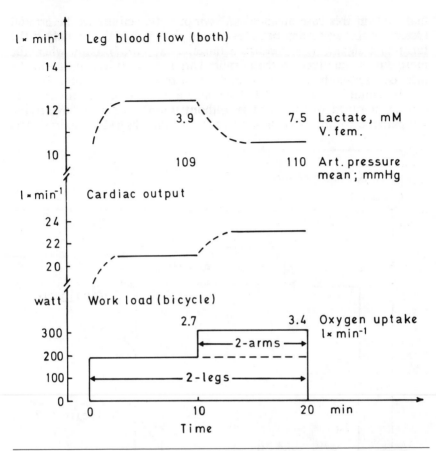

Figure 1.   Summary of results from a study by Secher, Clausen, and Klausen (1977). Please note that (a) the work load of the leg is kept constant through the experiment; (b) when the arms are added to the exercise the cardiac output increases somewhat, and the leg blood flow decreases simultaneously; and (c) this occurs without any change in blood pressure and in spite of an increase of the local vasodilator substances in the femoral vein.

This fact implies the need for a control system that during intense exercise with large muscle groups can produce vasoconstriction also of the vessels feeding heavily contracting muscles. If such a mechanism did not exist the blood pressure would drop. The control is mediated via the sympathetic nerves and the α-receptors of the arterial wall smooth muscles. These muscle cells are also affected by the composition of the arterial blood and by the interstitial ion and metabolite concentration. The net result, that is, the degree of vasodilation, depends on whether it is the local vasodilator substances or the sympathetic activity that has the greatest effect (Figure 2). When exercising with only a small muscle group, however intensely, the local vasodilating factors rule. It should be noted that even in this case an increased sympathetic activity to the arterial system of the exercising muscles is seen, but it has no (or only little) functional significance (Savard, Strange, et al., 1987). Only when the muscle mass involved in the exercise surpasses a critical limit will the increased sympathetic activity result in vasoconstriction (Table 3).

It cannot be stated exactly how large a fraction of the muscle mass can be involved in the exercise without interference from overriding sympathetic control. Calculations based on the observed maximal per-

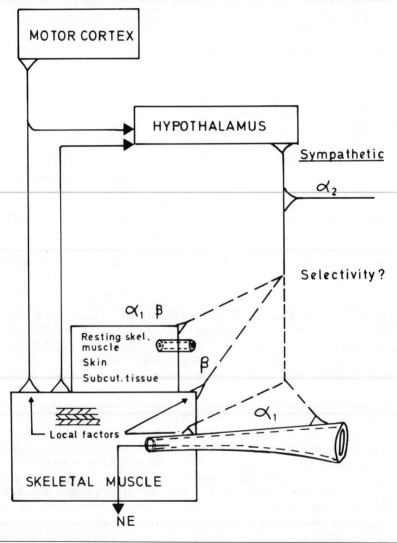

Figure 2.   A schematic illustration of the circulatory regulation (see text for details).

Table 3   Summary of Some Circulatory Variables and Norepinephrine Spillover From One Limb (Thigh)

	Cardiac output $1 \times min^{-1}$	Oxygen uptake $1 \times min^{-1}$	Leg blood flow $1 \times min^{-1}$	Norepinephrine[a] spillover $ng \times min^{-1}$
Rest	6.4	0.31	0.22	25
Knee extensor (1 leg)	10.4	1.1	5.25	250
Knee extensor (2 legs)	12.8	1.75	5.25	270
Knee extensor (1 leg) + 2 arms	15.0	2.42	4.9	480
Knee extensor (2 legs) + 2 arms	30.2	3.23	5.0	500
Knee extensor (2 legs)	—	2.24	6.80	370
Knee extensor (2 legs) + 2 arms	—	3.68	5.70	980

Note. The experiments were performed with a stepwise increase in the muscle mass involved in the exercise. NE spillover and limb blood flow were always measured over the same leg, which performed at the same work load.
[a] This is estimated from plasma flow, a-v_{fem} difference for norepinephrine and the extraction of norepinephrine based on ^{3H}NE turnover.

fusion data ($\approx 2 L \cdot kg^{-1} \cdot min^{-1}$; Saltin, 1985) for human skeletal muscles indicate that during exercise with one leg ($\approx 6-8$ kg muscles) the pump capacity of the heart is sufficient to produce an optimal flow. However, intense exercise with both legs ($\approx 12-16$ kg muscles) cannot be performed without some vasoconstriction in lower limb vessels because the peripheral conductance exceeds the pump capacity of the heart. These theoretical calculations are supported by experimental findings demonstrating that limb blood flow is higher during one-legged than during two-legged exercise (Klausen, Secher, Clausen, Hartling, & Trap-Jensen, 1982).

Similar calculations have been made for the rat (Mackie & Terjung, 1983). It was found that 70% to 80% of muscle mass has to be engaged in exercise to elicit maximal oxygen uptake. A difference between species is anticipated and should probably be viewed in light of the mass of muscle engaged in normal locomotion of the particular species. Humans moving in the upright posture have a lower heart capacity/muscular mass ratio than other mammals using four extremities and dependent upon their endurance capacity to survive (Table 4). Grande and Taylor (1965) have compiled data on heart weight in relation to body weight in a wide range of mammals. In humans the weight of the heart is only 0.3% to 0.4% of body weight, whereas it approaches 1% in dogs and horses (Table 4). The latter two species also have 2 to 3 times larger maximal oxygen uptake (100–160 ml · kg^{-1} · min^{-1}). Thus, in these species there is a more equal balance between the capacity of the heart to supply and the skeletal muscle to utilize oxygen. The miniature swine is in these respects most similar to humans.

The content of norepinephrine in plasma increases during exercise (Figure 3). From the preceding discussion it follows that the dominant fraction of the norepinephrine found in the blood during exercise originates from vessels in the skeletal muscles (Christensen et al., 1987; Savard et al., 1987). This agrees with the fact that the highest values are found when a very large muscle mass is engaged in the exercise (Holmqvist et al., 1986).

The crucial question is how the precise match between the output of the heart and the peripheral conductance is achieved (blood pressure maintained) during intense exercise with large muscle groups. The baroreceptors of the arterial system may play an important role. They may be so sensitive and respond so fast to pressure variations in the aorta and carotids that they can modulate peripheral conductance via the sympathetic nervous system by each heart beat. The ascending slope of the

Table 4   Summary of Some Variables Characterizing the Links in the Oxygen Transport of Humans and Some Other Species, as Well as Their Maximal Oxygen Uptake

	Heart weight (% of body weight)	Cardiac output (1 · min^{-1} · kg^{-1} BW)	Maximal oxygen uptake (ml · min^{-1} · kg^{-1} BW)
Humans	0.3/0.4	0.25/0.40	40/75
Pig (miniature swine)	0.5	0.40	60
Rat (lean)	0.6	0.50	75[a]
Dog (foxhounds)	0.8/0.9	0.80/0.90	120/145
Horse (standardbred)	0.8/0.9	0.70/0.90	120/150

Note. If two values are given, the second relates to the trained stage. Data in the above table are taken from Gleeson & Baldwin, 1981; Grande & Taylor, 1965; Mackie & Terjung, 1983; Musch, Haidet, Ordway, Longhurst, & Mitchell, 1985; Saltin & Åstrand, 1967; and Rose, personal communication.

[a] Values up to and just above 100 ml · kg^{-1} · min^{-1} have been reported.

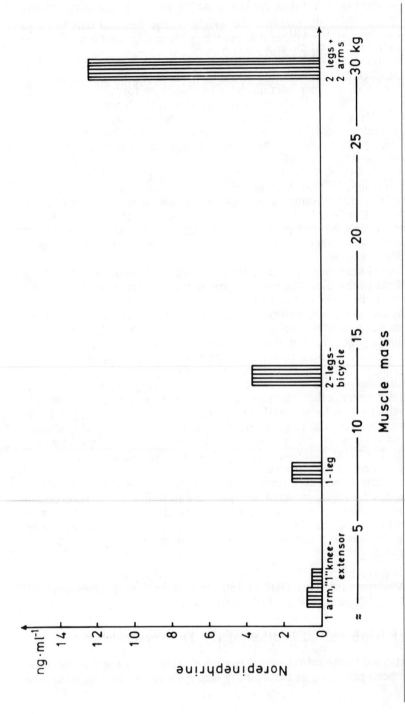

Figure 3.   The plasma norepinephrine concentration during exhausting exercise when different fractions of muscle mass are involved in the exercise. (Holmqvist et al., 1986; Lewis et al., 1983; Savard, Strange, Kiens, Saltin, Richter, & Christensen, 1987; Secher et al., 1977).

pressure wave may be less steep and the descending slope more steep when the ejected volume of the heart can barely fill a dilated peripheral bed. These subtle alterations in the form of the arterial pressure wave may be sensed by the baroreceptors and immediately cause adjustment of the peripheral resistance.

The question is whether the baroreceptors alone manage the regulation or whether receptors, for example in the heart, are also important. Experiments with hypervolemia during exercise performed by Kanstrup and Ekblom (1982) indicate that expanding blood volume by giving macrodex results in a somewhat increased stroke volume and cardiac output, which causes a small reduction in arterial pressure and an increased peripheral conductance. As the maximal heart rate for each individual is almost constant, the information on the distention of the heart ventricles (= end diastolic volume) may be the crucial variable for cardiac output. It might be that this variable determines the maximal allowable degree of vasodilation during exercise to exhaustion with a large fraction of the muscle mass. In line with this hypothesis is the finding that in dogs stroke volume and cardiac output during exhaustive running can become elevated when the pericardium is opened (Stray-Gundersen et al., 1986).

A simplification of this description is that the pump capacity of the heart determines the maximal oxygen uptake of the individual. This means that the kind of training that improves the pump capacity will also efficiently raise the individual's maximal aerobic capacity. However, this does not as a matter of course result in an optimally trained endurance capacity (see the following discussion). It does not seem to take a specific kind of training to increase the stroke volume or the maximal cardiac output. Training of high intensity with large muscle groups lasting some minutes gives a good result, and so does light training. The important difference is that when one is exercising at a low intensity, physical improvement calls for several hours of training each day throughout the week, whereas a similar improvement is attained in a considerably shorter period of time when previously sedentary men perform high intensity exercise. The long duration training may be efficient, however, in improving the endurance fitness.

Sedentary young men performing physical training during 3 months (Nordesjö, 1974) were grouped, and each group followed a strict protocol in regard to intensity and duration of the training as well as number of sessions per week. The brief summary illustrates three different training regimens, which all produced 15% to 20% improvement in maximal oxygen uptake.

1. Top intensity (HR ≈ 190 bpm), 15 min, once/week;
2. Moderate intensity (HR ≈ 150 bpm), 1 hr, 2 to 3 times/week;
3. Low intensity (HR ≈ 110 bpm), 2 hr, 5 times/week.

Peripheral Utilization of the Delivered Oxygen

As mentioned in the introduction, oxygen extraction by the skeletal muscles has been proposed as the limiting factor for maximal oxygen uptake

(Wagner, 1987; Wagner et al., 1986), which to some extent also is the conclusion of Di Prampero (1985) in his mathematical analysis of possible limitations to oxygen transport.

During bicycling or running, very little oxygen is left in femoral vein blood ($\approx$ 10–20 ml O_2 per liter blood), even during intense exhausting leg exercise (Table 5). This is the observation when blood is taken from a catheter placed distal to the saphenous vein. Not only the muscles, but also other tissues, including bone, connective tissues, and the skin, are drained. Blood from nonexercising muscles most likely has a relatively high content of oxygen. The blood flow measured in femoral vein is 6 to 8 L $\cdot$ min^{-1} during heavy exercise such as bicycling or running (Wahren, Saltin, Jorfeldt, & Pernow, 1974). If only 0.5 L $\cdot$ min^{-1} comes from tissues other than the contracting muscles, it can almost explain the oxygen observed in the vein draining the limb. Add to this the fact that even though the mitochondria need only a very small oxygen gradient ($\approx$ 0.5 mmHg between the outer membrane of the mitochondrial wall and the respiratory chain in order to saturate the latter with oxygen), a certain gradient is needed between the venous part of the capillaries and the mitochondria for a flux of oxygen to be present. Taking this into consideration and assuming that the oxygen tension is 2 mmHg at the venous end of the capillary, the amount of oxygen in the femoral vein can be explained. Thus, the oxygen extraction by contracting skeletal muscles is hardly a significant limiting factor for oxygen transport. Further, that the mitochondria in the skeletal muscles should restrain the oxygen utilization is even less likely.

It is noteworthy that some of the lowest pO_2 tensions are found when very physically inactive individuals exercise. This supports the notion that even a limited capillary network and a small mitochondrial volume in the skeletal muscles are sufficient for a complete oxygen utilization, provided that the mean transit time (MTT) is adequate. The need for a larger capillary network should be viewed with this in mind. As the muscle perfusion increases with endurance training, a more extensive capillary network is needed. The number of capillaries per mm^2 is approximately 280 in an untrained muscle, but 2 to 3 times higher in the

Table 5 Oxygen Tension and Content of Femoral Vein Blood During Exhaustive Leg Exercise

Physical condition	pO_2 (mmHg)	O_2 Content (ml $\cdot$ l^{-1})
Inactive	12	11
Sedentary	18	22
Some months training	10	18
Years training	8	10

most well-trained muscle (Table 6). It was earlier stated that the difference in maximal cardiac output between the completely untrained and the well-trained individual was almost the same. The maximal cardiac output in an untrained individual is approximately 20 L · min^{-1}, which during bicycling and running is distributed to the working legs ($\approx$ 16–17 L · min^{-1}) and to the rest of the body ($\approx$ 3–4 L · min^{-1}). The best endurance-trained individuals have a cardiac output of 35 to 40 L · min^{-1}, which renders over 30 to 35 L · min^{-1} to the leg muscles. Accordingly, maximal muscle perfusion in the muscles of the well-trained individual is proportionally larger, and add to this the larger capillary network. MTT might be around 1 s or less in the muscles involved in exercise (Saltin, 1985). As the capillary network seems to increase more than the maximal cardiac output (and maximal muscle perfusion) with endurance training, MTT is if anything longer in the muscles of the well-trained compared to the untrained individual during intense running or bicycling.

If only a small part of the muscle mass is engaged in the exercise, blood flow and oxygen uptake can markedly surpass the amount that can be extracted. An attempt to clarify this schematically is depicted in Figure 4. The larger the muscle blood flow, the larger the part of the muscle capillary network, and thus the capillary blood volume, that is utilized. When the network is utilized completely, MTT is reduced more markedly, and the oxygen content in the vein draining the muscle must also increase. That this indeed occurs when perfusion is excessive is seen in exercise with the knee extensors of only one leg. The a-v difference for oxygen over the exercising leg is only 110 to 120 ml · L^{-1}, compared with 160 to 170 ml · L^{-1} in normal bicycle exercise (Figure 5).

The Links and Capacity of the Respiratory Chain

By quantitating the amount of oxygen delivered to the muscles, which returns to the venous side of the systemic circulation, one can form a clear picture of where to find the most functionally significant changes

Table 6   Capillary Density in the Lateral Head of the Gastrocnemius Muscle in Physically Inactive Men and Endurance Athletes

	Cap. per mm^2	Cap. around			Cap. per fiber
		ST	FT$_a$	FT$_b$	
Inactive men	280	2.8	2.6	2.2	0.8
Sedentary men	320	3.0	2.8	2.6	1.1
Marathoners	680	6.8	6.5	(6.4)	3.2
Cross-country skiers	720	7.4	7.0	(7.0)	3.4

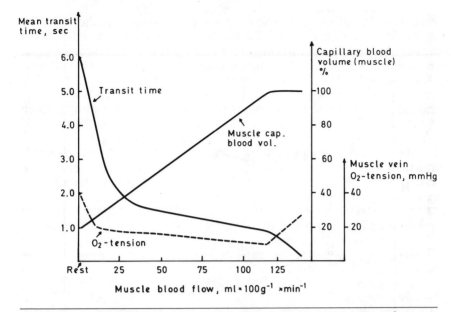

Figure 4. A schematic attempt to illustrate how the oxygen content of venous blood from a contracting muscle might increase during very intense exercise. The explanation might be that when the blood flow surpasses a critical level, the entire capillary network is utilized, whereafter an increased flow results in a markedly lowered mean transit time.

related to training status (Figure 6). To each kilogram of muscle 160 to 170 ml O_2 per minute is delivered, and of this only about 10 ml is not "used" during maximal exercise. This applies to a very physically inactive individual. A sedentary individual can deliver some more oxygen ($\approx$ 220 ml $\cdot$ kg^{-1} $\cdot$ min^{-1}). The amount of oxygen delivered to the muscle is further enhanced with endurance training and reaches 400 to 450 ml $\cdot$ kg^{-1} $\cdot$ min^{-1} in the most well-trained individuals. In their femoral vein blood "only" 10 to 15 ml O_2 $\cdot$ kg^{-1} $\cdot$ min^{-1} remains. Maximal delivery of oxygen to muscles in humans during exercise is closely linked with the maximal cardiac output. Thus, the variable that varies the most is the delivery of oxygen to the muscle, which from a functional standpoint must be regarded as the most crucial factor setting the upper limit for the aerobic capacity of the individual.

The amount of oxygen that can be transported to the skeletal muscles can now be defined more precisely (Table 7). From the data of Dempsey (1986); Dempsey, Hanson, and Henriksson (1984); and others (Rowell et al., 1964, Terrados, Mizuno, & Andersen, 1985), it appears that the maximal oxygen transfer capacity of the lung is around 80 to 100 ml O_2 per kilogram body weight and minutes (ml $\cdot$ kg^{-1} $\cdot$ min^{-1}). Endurance training can to a slight extent affect this capacity of the lungs. In an untrained individual the heart can produce a systemic oxygen transport

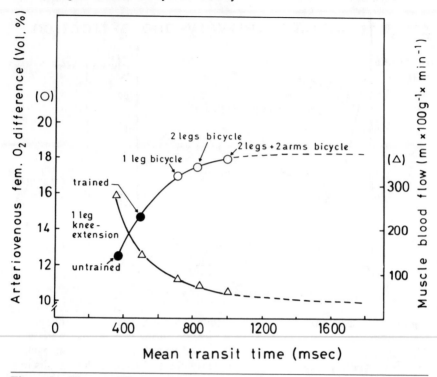

Figure 5. The a-v difference for oxygen over an exercising extremity when different combinations of muscle synergies are involved in the exercise. The given mean transit times are estimated (Andersen & Saltin, 1985; Saltin et al., 1968; Saltin et al., 1976; Secher et al., 1977).

of around 40 to 50 ml $\cdot$ kg^{-1} $\cdot$ min^{-1}. In contrast to the lungs the capacity of the heart is trainable and can reach a value equal to or higher than the capacity of the lungs.

The peripheral circulatory network of the muscles is capable of receiving a flow corresponding to 300 to 400 ml O_2 $\cdot$ kg^{-1} (muscle) $\cdot$ min^{-1} (Andersen & Saltin, 1985; Saltin et al., 1986). From these studies we also know that at least 300 ml O_2 $\cdot$ kg^{-1} (muscle) $\cdot$ min^{-1} can be utilized by the muscle. This applies for a muscle not especially trained. Very well-trained muscles can receive a blood flow corresponding to 500 to 600 ml O_2 $\cdot$ kg^{-1} (muscle) $\cdot$ min^{-1} or more, and most of the oxygen can also be utilized. Thus, this summary shows that the pump capacity of the heart is the limiting factor in the transport of oxygen. This applies for untrained as well as for the very best endurance-trained individuals, although in some of the latter the upper capacity of the lungs to transfer oxygen has also been reached.

Recently Dempsey (1986) came to a somewhat different conclusion, in which the limiting factors to oxygen uptake were the muscles and the heart of the untrained individual rather than the capacity of the lungs.

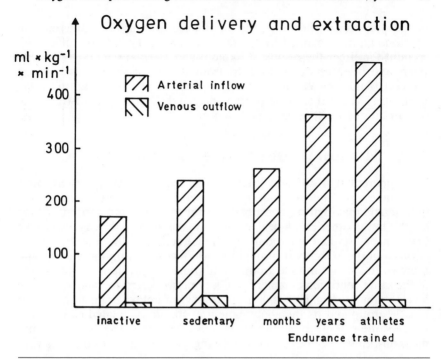

Figure 6. Attempts are made to calculate the oxygen delivery to 1 kg of exercising muscles and the amount of oxygen left in the vein draining the working extremity. (Saltin, 1969; Saltin et al., 1968).

Table 7   Summary of the Capacity to Transport Oxygen (ml · kg⁻¹ · min⁻¹) Via the Lungs and Cardiovascular System to its Utilization in the Muscle

	Sedentary individuals	Athletes
Upper limit of the lungs to transfer oxygen	80–100	80–100
Upper limit of the heart to deliver oxygen (per kg body weight)	40–50	80–100
Upper limit of the muscle to consume oxygen (per kg muscles)	300–400	>500

In the well-trained, however, the lungs were limiting. The difference in opinion can be explained by the fact that Dempsey did not sufficiently account for either the results of Ekblom and Hermansen (1968) on elite skiers and orienteers or the results from studies of small muscle group exercise (Andersen & Saltin, 1985; Rowell et al., 1986; Saltin, 1985; Wesche, 1981). If these results are considered, Dempsey's illustration of the conditions must be modified (Figure 7).

Maximal Oxygen Uptake—Endurance Fitness

It is apparent that different links in the oxygen transport system limit maximal oxygen uptake, peak oxygen uptake, and endurance. In healthy individuals maximal oxygen uptake is set by the pump capacity of the heart. On the other hand, peak oxygen uptake, that is, the oxygen uptake that can be attained when only a minor fraction of the muscle mass is engaged in the exercise, is limited by local factors within the muscle, and more so in smaller muscle groups. Endurance performance is a function of the same conditions, namely capillary network and metabolic enzyme levels in the muscle. Hence, both peak oxygen uptake of an extremity or muscle group and its metabolic potential should be related closely, and to the same extent, to endurance (Kiens & Terrados, personal communication). In whole body exercise (rowing, cross-country skiing, or swim-

UNTRAINED $(40\,ml \times kg^{-1} \times min^{-1})$
TRAINED $(80\,ml \times kg^{-1} \times min^{-1})$

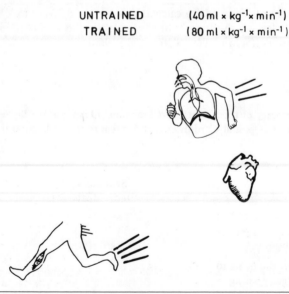

Figure 7.   Schematic illustration (modified from Dempsey, 1986) of the main limiting link(s) in sedentary and trained individuals. In the sedentary individual the pump capacity of the heart has the lowest capacity. After very extensive endurance exercise the pump capacity approaches the capacity of the lungs, which is influenced by training only to a minor extent.

ming) or two-legged exercise (bicycling or running), endurance may relate more to the local training status of the involved muscles than to maximal oxygen uptake. This latter point is well documented in rats, where the endurance capacity was closely matched with the mitochondrial enzyme levels in leg muscles, but not equally well with the maximal oxygen uptake (Davies, Packer, & Brooks, 1981).

In humans, similar observations are most easily obtained during detraining, when a dissociation is found between the rate of fall in maximal oxygen uptake and muscle enzyme levels: The former variable is maintained fairly well over some weeks in spite of no training, whereas the mitochondrial volume quickly returns to pretraining level. If endurance tests are performed when this discrepancy between maximal oxygen uptake and local muscle enzyme capacity is at its largest, one can observe a marked reduction in performance. Under more ordinary circumstances, it is not so easy to demonstrate that maximal oxygen uptake and endurance fitness may not be directly coupled. This is because the muscle adaptation rather closely varies with an individual's maximal oxygen uptake. In upper body exercise of sedentary subjects, endurance performance is considerably lower than when lower limbs perform at the same relative work intensity (Falkel, Sawka, Levine, Pimental, & Pandolf, 1986; Pimental, Sawka, Billings, & Trad, 1984). This is most likely a reflection of an "overperfusion" of arm muscles during arm work relative to their mass when compared to leg muscles, which may relate to the elevated blood pressure observed during arm exercise (Clausen, Klausen, Rasmussen, & Trap-Jensen, 1973; Stenberg, Åstrand, Ekblom, Royce, & Saltin, 1967). Thus, the measured peak VO_2 of this muscle mass is somewhat higher than it should be relative to its "trained status"; that is, the upper body is most commonly "sedentary" relative to the lower body musculature, and endurance time is correspondingly shortened (Falkel et al., 1986).

One aspect of endurance fitness that puzzles many is that it can be altered by a factor of 2 to 4, whereas maximal oxygen uptake usually only varies by 20% to 50%. The explanation, in part, is given in Figure 8. Endurance time is a function of the relative work intensity and increases exponentially with decreasing relative exercise rate. Hence, if maximal oxygen uptake is increased by 20%, a work rate demanding 90% of maximal oxygen uptake before training represents "only" a relative work intensity of 70% after the training, and endurance time can be expected to increase by a factor of five or more (Figure 8). The amount of energy utilized increases in a similar fashion. The ability to perform longer at the same relative exercise intensity can also be improved with endurance training, but the magnitude of this change is minor. These relationships are clearly demonstrated in work by Costill, Branam, Eddy, and Sparks (1971) and Costill, Thomason, and Roberts (1973) of English long distance runners. The speed at which the runners ran a 10-mi (16-km) race was related primarily to the maximal oxygen uptake, which varied between 55 ml and 82 ml $\cdot$ kg^{-1} $\cdot$ min^{-1}, whereas all ran at very similar relative exercise intensities, (i.e., between 82% and 92%), and no

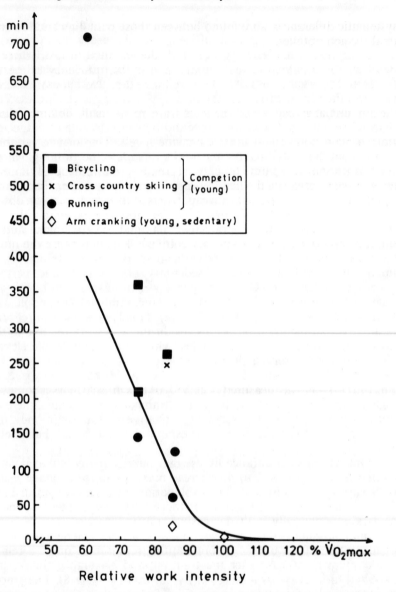

Figure 8. The relationship between the relative work load (oxygen uptake in percent of maximal oxygen uptake) and time to exhaustion in well-trained individuals (continuous line). The other symbols indicate data on elite athletes during competition, where oxygen uptake has been measured (filled symbols). Unfilled symbols denote arm cranking (for references see Savard, Kiens, & Saltin, 1987).

systematic differences were found between those with high and low maximal oxygen uptakes.

It has therefore been suggested that whereas speed or work intensity is set by the maximal oxygen uptake and by the efficiency in the task performed (energy economy), the time this speed can be maintained is more a function of the efficiency in usage of the glycogen stores. Thus, the amount of glycogen and the local training status of the limb muscles engaged in the exercise are decisive for the maintenance of a certain relative work intensity, which, in turn, is well correlated to measured levels of blood lactate at given running speeds. It is possible to train various muscle groups of the body separately and thereby enhance the peak oxygen uptake of the muscle as well as its endurance capacity without improving the central cardiovascular capacity and maximal oxygen uptake (Gaffney, Grimby, Danneskiold-Samsøe, & Halskov, 1981). This extends to the training of one leg or each leg separately, where only a small effect on the maximal oxygen uptake has been observed even though the peak oxygen uptake and endurance capacity of the trained leg has improved (Klausen et al., 1982; Saltin et al., 1976).

Acknowledgments

Studies performed in this laboratory were supported by the Danish Heart Association and the Research Council of the Danish Sports Federation.

References

Andersen, P., Adams, R.P., Sjøgaard, G., Thorboe, A., & Saltin, B. (1985). Dynamic knee extension as a model for the study of an isolated exercising muscle in man. *Journal of Applied Physiology, 59*, 1647–1653.

Andersen, P., & Saltin, B. (1985). Maximal perfusion of skeletal muscle in man. *Journal of Physiology, 366*, 233–249.

Armstrong, R.B., Delp, M.D., Goljan, E.F., & Laughlin, M.H. (1987). Distribution of blood flow in muscles of miniature swine during exercise. *Journal of Applied Physiology, 62*, 1285–1298.

Blomqvist, C.G., & Saltin, B. (1983). Cardiovascular adaptations to physical training. *Annual Review of Physiology, 45*, 169–189.

Christensen, N.J., Kiens, B., Richter, E.A., Saltin, B., Savard, G., & Strange, S. (1987). Noradrenaline spillover from skeletal muscle during exercise at various intensities in man. *Journal of Physiology, 390*, 252P.

Clausen, J.P., Klausen, K., Rasmussen, B., & Trap-Jensen, J. (1973). Central and peripheral circulatory changes after training of the arms or legs. *American Journal of Physiology, 225*, 675–682.

Costill, D.L., Branam, G., Eddy, D., & Sparks, K. (1971). Determinants of marathon running success. *Internationale Zeitschrift für Angewandte Physiologie, 29*, 249–254.

Costill, D.L., Thomason, H., & Roberts, E. (1973). Fractional utilization of the aerobic capacity during distance running. *Medicine and Science in Sports, 5*, 248–252.

Davies, K.J.A., Packer, L., & Brooks, G.A. (1981). Biochemical adaptations of mitochondria, muscle and whole-animal respiration to endurance training. *Archives Biochemica & Biophysica 1981,* **209,** 539–554.

Dempsey, J.A. (1986). Is the lung built for exercise? *Medicine and Science in Sports and Exercise,* **18,** 143–155.

Dempsey, J.A., Hanson, P.G., & Henriksson, K.S. (1984). Exercise-induced arterial hypoxemia in healthy persons at sea level. *Journal of Physiology,* **355,** 161–175.

Di Prampero, P. (1985). Metabolic and circulatory limitations to $\dot{V}O_2$max at the whole animal level. *Journal of Experimental Biology,* **115,** 319–331.

Ekblom, B., & Hermansen, L. (1968). Cardiac output in athletes. *Journal of Applied Physiology,* **25,** 619–625.

Falkel, J.E., Sawka, M.N., Levine, L., Pimental, N.A., & Pandolf, K.B. (1986). Upper-body exercise performance: Comparison between women and men. *Ergonomics,* **29,** 145–154.

Gaffney, F.A., Grimby, G., Danneskiold-Samsøe, B., & Halskov, O. (1981). Adaptation to peripheral muscle training. *Scandinavian Journal of Rehabilitation Medicine,* **13,** 1–6.

Gleeson, T.T., & Baldwin, K.M. (1981). Cardiovascular response to treadmill exercise in untrained rats. *Journal of Applied Physiology,* **50,** 1206–1211.

Grande, F., & Taylor, H.L. (1965). Adaptive changes in the heart, vessels, and patterns of control under chronically high loads. In W.F. Hamilton & P. Dow (Eds.), *Handbook of physiology: Circulation* (Vol. 3, pp. 2615–2678). Washington, DC: American Physiological Society.

Holmgren, A., & Åstrand, P.-O. (1966). D_L and the dimensions and functional capacities of the O_2 transport system in humans. *Journal of Applied Physiology,* **21,** 1463–1470.

Holmqvist, N., Secher, N.H., Sander-Jensen, K., Knigge, U., Warberg, J., & Schwartz, T.W. (1986). Sympathoadrenal and parasympathetic responses to exercise. *Journal of Sports Sciences,* **4,** 123–128.

Kanstrup, I.-L. & Ekblom, B. (1982). Acute hypervolemia, cardiac performance, and aerobic power during exercise. *Journal of Applied Physiology, Respiratory, Environmental and Exercise Physiology,* **52,** 1186–1191.

Klausen, K., Secher, N.H., Clausen, J.P., Hartling, D., & Trap-Jensen, J. (1982). Control and regional circulatory adaptations to one-leg training. *Journal of Applied Physiology,* **52,** 976–983.

Lewis, S.F., Taylor, W.F., Graham, R.M., Pettinger, W.A., Schutte, J.E., & Blomqvist, O.G. (1983). Cardiovascular responses to exercise as functions of absolute and relative work load. *Journal of Applied Physiology,* **54,** 1314–1323.

Mackie, B.G., & Terjung, R.L. (1983). Blood flow to different skeletal muscle fiber types during contractions. *American Journal of Physiology,* **245,** H264–H275.

Musch, T.I., Haidet, G.C., Ordway, G.A., Longhurst, J.C., & Mitchell, J.H. (1985). Dynamic exercise training in foxhounds. I. Oxygen consumption and hemodynamic responses. *Journal of Applied Physiology,* **59,** 183–189.

Nordesjö, L.-O. (1974). The effect of quantitated training of the capacity for short and prolonged work. *Acta Physiologica Scandinavica,* **90** (Suppl. 405).

Pimental, N.A., Sawka, M.N., Billings, D.S., & Trad, L.A. (1984). Physiological responses to prolonged upper-body exercise. *Medicine and Science in Sports and Exercise,* **16,** 360–365.

Rowell, L.B., Saltin, B., Kiens, B., & Christensen, N.J. (1986). Is peak quadriceps blood flow in humans even higher during exercise with hypoxia? *American Journal of Physiology,* **251,** H1038–H1044.

Rowell, L.B., Taylor, H.L., Wang, Y., & Carlson, W.B. (1964). Saturation of arterial blood with oxygen during maximal exercise. *Journal of Applied Physiology,* **19,** 284–286.

Saltin, B. (1969). Physiological effects of physical conditioning. *Medicine & Science in Sports,* **1,** 50–56.

Saltin, B. (1985). Hemodynamic adaptations to exercise. *American Journal of Cardiology,* **55,** 42D–47D.

Saltin, B., & Åstrand, P.-O. (1967). Maximal oxygen uptake in athletes. *Journal of Applied Physiology,* **23,** 353–358.

Saltin, B., Blomqvist, G., Mitchell, J.H., Johnson, R.L., Jr., Wildenthal, K., & Chapman, C.B. (1968). Response to exercise after bed rest and after training. *Circulation,* **38,** 1–78.

Saltin, B., Kiens, B., Savard, G.K., & Pedersen, P.K. (1986). Role of hemoglobin and capillarization for oxygen delivery and extraction in muscular exercise. *Acta Physiologica Scandinavica,* **128,** 21–32.

Saltin, B., Nazar, K., Costill, D.L., Stein, E., Jansson, E., Essen, B., & Gollnick, P.D. (1976). The nature of the training response; peripheral and central adaptations to one-legged exercise. *Acta Physiologica Scandinavica,* **96** 289–305.

Savard, G., Kiens, B., & Saltin, B. (1987). Central cardiovascular factors as limits to endurance; with a note on the distinction between maximal oxygen uptake and endurance fitness. In D. Macleod, R. Maughan, M. Nimmo, R. Reilly, & C. Williams (Eds.), *Exercise: benefits, limits and adaptations* (pp. 162–180). London: E. & F.N. Spon.

Savard, G., Strange, S., Kiens, B., Saltin, B., Richter, E.A., & Christensen, N.J. (1987). Norepinephrine spillover during exercise in active versus resting skeletal muscle in man. *Acta Physiologica Scandinavica,* **131,** 507–515.

Secher, N.H., Clausen, J.P., & Klausen, K. (1977). Central and regional circulatory effects of adding arm exercise to leg exercise. *Acta Physiologica Scandinavica,* **100,** 288–297.

Stenberg, J., Åstrand, P.-O., Ekblom, B., Royce, J., & Saltin, B. (1967). Hemodynamic response to work with different muscle groups, sitting and supine. *Journal of Applied Physiology,* **22,** 61–70.

Stray-Gundersen, J., Musch, T.I., Haidet, G.C., Swain, D.P., Ordway, G.A., & Mitchell, J.H. (1986). The effect of pericardiectomy on maximal oxygen consumption and maximal cardiac output in untrained dogs. *Circulation Research,* **58,** 523-530.

Terrados, N., Mizuno, M., & Andersen, H. (1985). Reduction in maximal oxygen uptake at low altitudes; role of training status and lung function. *Clinical Physiology,* **5,** 75-79.

Wagner, P.D. (1988). Tissue diffusion limitation of maximal O_2 and effluent muscle venous pO_2. In J.R. Sutton, C.S. Houston, & G. Coates (Eds.), *Hypoxia: The tolerable limits* (pp. 44-51). Indianapolis: Benchmark.

Wagner, P.D., Reeves, J.T., Sutton, J.R., Cymerman, A., Groves, B.M., Calconian, M.K., & Young, P.M. (1986). Possible limitations of maximal O_2 uptake by peripheral tissue diffusion. *Annual Review of Respiratory Diseases,* **133,** A202.

Wahren, J., Saltin, B., Jorfeldt, L., & Pernow, B. (1974). Influence of age on the local circulatory adaptation to leg exercise. *Scandinavian Journal of Clinical Laboratory Investigation,* **33,** 79-86.

Wesche, J. (1986). The time course and magnitude of blood flow changes in the human quadriceps muscles following isometric contraction. *Journal of Physiology,* **377,** 445-463.

Hormonal Adaptations to Exercise Training

Erik A. Richter

August Krogh Institute
Copenhagen, Denmark

Exercise is the most powerful physiologic perturbation experienced by healthy humans. It requires major metabolic and cardiovascular adjustments to increase the supply of oxygen and fuels to the working muscles while maintaining oxygen and fuel delivery to the vital organs. To accomplish this task, changes in autonomic nervous activity and in hormone secretion occur during exercise. The rather sharp distinction between the nervous system and the hormonal system that was customary until recently is no longer possible because substances earlier considered genuine hormones may be released from nerves (e.g., insulin, gastrin), and neurotransmitters may spill over into the blood and act as hormones (e.g., norepinephrine). Therefore, in this review, no sharp distinction between autonomic nervous and hormonal adaptation to exercise training will be made.

A single bout of exercise is characterized by increased plasma concentrations of a large variety of hormones and decreased concentrations of only a few hormones. Although only some hormones have been studied, the general impression is that large changes in hormone concentrations during exercise are the result mainly of changes in secretion rate rather than changes in clearance, although clearance for the many hormones that are degraded primarily in the liver may be expected to decrease during exercise as splanchnic blood flow decreases (Galbo, 1986). A key role in the neuroendocrine response to exercise is increased sympathoadrenal activity, but also occurring are increased secretion of adrenocortotropic hormone (ACTH) and cortisol; of renin, angiotensin, and aldosterone; and of growth hormone (GH) and glucagon; and decreased secretion of insulin. However, the role of these latter hormones does not seem to be as important for regulation of circulation and metabolism during exercise. The plasma concentration of many other peptides and hormones also changes during exercise; however, it is beyond the scope of this review to go into any detail as regards stimuli for changes in secretion of the various hormones, changes in secretion during various

25

kinds of exercise, and so on. Instead the reader is referred to a recent review on the topic (Galbo).

This review will describe changes in neuroendocrine activity at rest and during exercise as well as changes in target tissue sensitivity induced by endurance training. Furthermore, some attention will be given to the functional significance of the altered neuroendocrine status in the trained state.

Hormonal Changes at Rest

Norepinephrine

Conflicting results exist regarding whether endurance training decreases the activity in the sympathetic nervous system at rest. The question has been addressed most often by measuring plasma norepinephrine concentration, assuming that it correlates well with overall sympathetic activity. In fact, fairly good correlations have been found between plasma norepinephrine concentration and directly recorded sympathetic activity in the peroneal nerve (Wallin et al., 1981). However, it should be emphasized that the sympathetic activity can be very differentiated (Mitchell, Kaufman, & Iwamoto, 1983; Savard et al., 1987); hence changes in nerve traffic to one organ need not be reflected in measurable changes in plasma norepinephrine concentrations in arterial or mixed venous blood. Nevertheless, when endurance-trained athletes were compared with untrained subjects, no differences in resting plasma norepinephrine concentrations were found (Kjær, Christensen, Sonne, Richter, & Galbo, 1985; Kjær, Farrell, Christensen, & Galbo, 1986; Kjær et al., 1984; Lehmann, Dickhuth, Schmid, Porzig, & Keul, 1984; Svedenhag, 1985). Peripheral sympathetic nervous activity measured directly by nerve recording (Figure 1) was found to be unrelated to training status (Svedenhag, Wallin, Sundlöf, & Henriksson, 1984).

In previously untrained subjects 4 months of endurance training, which increased VO_2max by 18%, did not significantly decrease resting plasma norepinephrine concentrations (Svedenhag, 1985). Similar findings in short-term training studies in which comparable increases in VO_2max were obtained have been described by others (Hartley et al., 1972; Koivisto, Hendler, Nadel, & Felig, 1982; Winder, Hagberg, Hickson, Ehsani, & McLane, 1978). However, a decrease in resting plasma norepinephrine concentrations as well as in sympathetic nervous activity (as reflected by whole body norepinephrine spillover, which is the average rate at which norepinephrine released from sympathetic nerves enters plasma) was found in 10 out of 12 subjects after 4 weeks of hard endurance training (Jennings et al., 1986). Furthermore, in that study resting mean blood pressure decreased due to a decrease in total peripheral resistance in all 12 subjects.

Epinephrine

As regards the plasma concentration of epinephrine at rest, longitudinal training studies have shown that there is no effect from endurance training

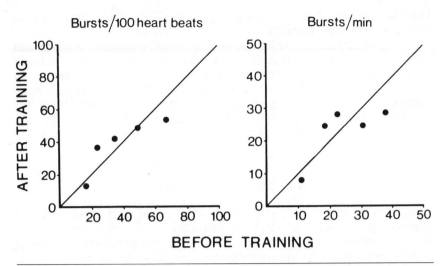

Figure 1. Muscle sympathetic nervous activity in the peroneal nerve in 5 subjects before and after 8 weeks of training. From "Skeletal Muscle Sympathetic Activity at Rest in Trained and Untrained Subjects" by J. Svedenhag, B.G. Wallin, G. Sundlöf, and J. Henriksson, 1984, *Acta Physiologica Scandinavica,* **120,** 499–504. Reprinted by permission.

(Hartley et al., 1972; Jennings et al., 1986; Koivisto et al., 1982; Lehmann et al., 1984; Svedenhag, 1985; Winder et al., 1978). However, in athletes who have been training for years, it has been found that plasma concentration of epinephrine at rest is increased compared with controls (Kjær et al., 1984, 1985, 1986). Thus, it may be that years of training induces adaptations in the adrenal gland that are not found in longitudinal studies over only a few months.

Other Hormones

Plasma concentrations of other hormones may be changed by training. For instance, the plasma concentration of insulin is lower in well-trained than in untrained subjects (Kjær et al., 1986; Wirth et al., 1981). Furthermore, in highly trained male runners, the resting evening plasma concentration of ACTH and cortisol was elevated compared to less-trained and untrained subjects, and the response to ovine corticotropin-releasing hormone was also diminished in the well-trained subjects, suggesting impairment of the hypothalamic-pituitary-adrenal axis (Luger et al., 1987). A difference in plasma cortisol concentration at rest (in the morning) between athletes and untrained subjects, however, was not found by Kjær et al. (1986) or by Hackney, Sinning, and Bruot (1988).

In males, a program of endurance training does not change resting levels of testosterone (Kuoppasalmi, Näveri, Kosunen, Härkönen, & Adlercreutz, 1981). However, in male endurance-trained athletes testosterone and free testosterone were lower and luteinizing hormone (LH) higher than in sedentary controls (Hackney et al., 1988). These findings thus suggest that in endurance-trained athletes, gonadal and not pituitary function may be impaired. The finding of changed hormonal status in athletes endurance-trained for years but no such changes in untrained subjects undergoing only months of training suggest that long-term endocrine adaptations to years of endurance training take place. Another possibility is of course that the athletes are differently genetically equipped than the untrained controls. Changes in gonadotropin and sex steroid secretion may be found in endurance-trained women, as described later in this review.

Functional Significance

The effect of exercise training on blood pressure (and presumably on sympathetic nervous activity) has attracted considerable interest as a possible means of treatment of mild hypertension. Several studies in mildly to moderately hypertensive patients have found a decrease in mean arterial blood pressure of 5 to 10 mmHg after training, but many studies have methodological problems that bring into question the conclusions (for review, see Seals & Hagberg, 1984). However, even a single bout of exercise may lower blood pressure for hours (Fitzgerald, 1981; Wilcox, Bennett, Brown, & MacDonald, 1982). In a recent well-controlled study, 3 and 7 weeks of endurance training in mildly hypertensive patients decreased plasma norepinephrine concentration as well as total peripheral resistance and blood pressure (Nelson, Jennings, Esler, & Korner, 1986). Thus, there is evidence for a decrease in norepinephrine concentration and blood pressure in hypertensive patients following endurance training.

The functional significance of changes in plasma concentrations of epinephrine, testosterone, LH, and (in some studies) ACTH at rest is not readily apparent. In fact there may be none, or if any it may be more deleterious than beneficial. It should, however, be realized that the observed hormonal changes between endurance-trained athletes and untrained controls represent differences obtained in highly selected subgroups of the population. However, the findings do raise the question of whether the described hormonal changes seen in athletes compared to untrained controls actually indicate that many years of hard endurance training impose considerable stress on the body that—at least for some body functions—may be more harmful than beneficial.

Hormonal Changes During Exercise

The plasma concentration of the catecholamines increases during exercise depending on the relative exercise intensity (for references see Galbo, 1986; Svedenhag, 1985). Because after endurance training the same absolute work load will be a lesser relative work load, it follows that the plasma concentration of the catecholamines during exercise at a fixed work load decreases after training (Hartley et al., 1972; Svedenhag, 1985;

Winder et al., 1978; Winder, Hickson, Hagberg, Ehsani, & McLane, 1979). It has even been described that during prolonged low intensity exercise at the same relative work load, the plasma concentration of the catecholamines was decreased after 6 weeks of endurance training (Koivisto et al., 1982). Surprisingly, the adaptation can be found after only one week of training (Figure 2) and seems to be essentially completed after only 3 weeks (Winder et al., 1978). The rapidity and magnitude of adaptation are probably dependent upon the intensity and frequency of training, but it is interesting that the hormonal adaptation occurs much more rapidly than the increase in VO_2max. Thus, the adaptation cannot be elicited solely by changes in relative work load.

In contrast to these findings obtained before and after a rather short training period, cross-sectional studies by Kjær et al. (1986) have provided data that suggest that many years of hard endurance training may result in adaptations different from those found after only a few months of training. Thus, at the same absolute submaximal work load the epinephrine concentration in plasma was similar in athletes and in controls in spite of markedly lower norepinephrine concentrations in the former. Furthermore, it has been reported that during maximal and "supramaximal" exercise the epinephrine but not the norepinephrine response was significantly larger in athletes than in sedentary controls (Kjær et al., 1986). These findings may reflect the development of a higher maximum epinephrine secretion rate by endurance-trained athletes. Further support for this concept has recently been published (Kjær & Galbo, 1988). Although these athletes may be genetically predisposed with a large capacity to secrete epinephrine, it is a fascinating idea that neuroendocrine tissue, like muscle, may adapt to frequent use. Following training, other hormones are also found in lower concentrations in plasma during exercise at a given absolute work load; for instance, ACTH (Buono, Yeager, & Sucec, 1987) and glucagon (Koivisto et al., 1982).

Functional Significance

The functional significance of the training-induced decrease in plasma concentrations of the catecholamines and glucagon found during submaximal exercise is readily apparent when one views the hormonal response to exercise as a mechanism promoting fuel delivery (primarily of carbohydrate) to the working muscles. Thus, following training, when the muscle is able to rely more on fat combustion than before training, the need for mobilization of carbohydrate stores is less, and consequently the hormonal response is decreased. It is in line with this thinking that the epinephrine and glucagon response to exercise is determined to a large extent by the plasma glucose concentration; thus secretion of these hormones is exaggerated when the plasma glucose concentration falls (see Galbo, 1986). As regards the apparent increased ability of endurance-trained athletes to achieve a higher rate of epinephrine secretion during high intensity exercise, this adaptation may be regarded as making athletes better fit to sustain such bursts of intense activity.

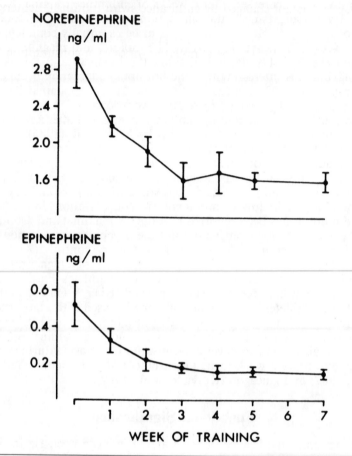

CATECHOLAMINE CONC. AFTER
5 MIN AT 1500 KPM · MIN⁻¹

NOREPHRINE
ng / ml

EPINEPHRINE
ng / ml

WEEK OF TRAINING

Figure 2.   Plasma catecholamines after 5 min exercise at the same absolute work load before and after training for 1 to 7 weeks. From "Time Course of Sympathoadrenal Adaptation to Endurance Exercise Training in Man" by W.W. Winder, J.M. Hagberg, R.C. Hickson, A.A. Ehsani, and J.A. McLane, 1978, *Journal of Applied Physiology, 45,* 370–374. Reprinted by permission.

Changes in Hormone Sensitivity of Target Tissues

Sensitivity to Catecholamines

Hormonal adaptations to exercise training also relate to possible training-induced changes in hormone sensitivity of target tissues. For instance, the action of epinephrine is enhanced in adipocytes from trained subjects

(Crampes, Beauville, Riviere, & Garrigues, 1986) and rats (Bukowiecki et al., 1980; Williams & Bishop, 1982). However, epinephrine-stimulated production of cyclic adenosine monophosphate (cyclic AMP) in perfused rat muscle was not changed by endurance swim training (Richter, Kjær, & Galbo, 1986), even though others have found an increase in beta-adrenergic receptors in muscle following training by running (Williams, Caron, & Daniel, 1984). The stimulation of oxygen consumption by ep-inephrine (probably primarily an alpha-adrenergic response [Richter, Ruderman, & Galbo, 1982]) was, however, enhanced in perfused hind-limbs from trained compared with untrained rats (Richter, Christensen, Ploug, & Galbo, 1984).

Sensitivity to Insulin

Exercise training has been shown to diminish the increase in plasma insulin concentration in response to a glucose load in both humans (Lohmann, Liebold, Heilmann, Senger, & Pohl, 1978; Rodnick, Haskell, Swislocki, Foley, & Reaven, 1987) and rat (Berger et al., 1979). Nevertheless, glucose tolerance is unchanged or improved (Berger et al.; Lohmann et al; Rodnick et al.). These findings indicate that insulin action is enhanced in the trained state. This assumption has been directly confirmed using the euglycemic insulin clamp procedure (James, Kraegen, & Chisholm, 1985; Rodnick et al.). The tissues involved include adipose tissue (Craig, Hammons, Garthwaite, Jarett, & Holloszy, 1981; James et al.; Rodnick et al.; Vinten & Galbo, 1983), possibly liver (Rodnick et al.), and, probably more important, skeletal muscle (James et al.; Mondon, Dolkas, & Reaven, 1980). Interestingly, the endocrine pancreas apparently adapts to the increased peripheral insulin sensitivity by being less responsive to hyperglycemia. Thus, during similar levels of sustained hyperglycemia, insulin secretion in trained subjects is markedly lower than in untrained subjects (King et al., 1987; Mikines et al., 1987) (Figure 3).

Skeletal muscle is the largest consumer of glucose during a glucose challenge. Therefore changes in insulin sensitivity of muscle due to training are important on the whole body level. It appears that the level of habitual physical activity markedly influences insulin action in skeletal muscle. Thus, insulin action in muscles is increased in trained compared to untrained rats (James et al., 1985; Mondon et al., 1980); in trained humans, whole body glucose uptake (thought to reflect mainly uptake in muscle) during euglycemic hyperinsulinemia is increased compared with untrained subjects (King et al., 1987; Mikines et al., 1987; Rodnick et al., 1987). Conversely, decreased levels of activity impair insulin action in muscle, and the effect seems to be at least primarily localized to the muscles involved. Thus, when normal volunteers had the knee joint of one leg immobilized by a splint for only 7 days, insulin action on thigh glucose uptake during euglycemic hyperinsulinemia was decreased compared with the nonimmobilized leg (Table 1). Similarly, in rodents limb

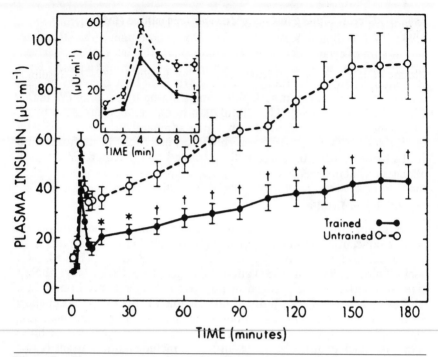

Figure 3. Plasma concentrations of insulin in trained and untrained subjects during a hyperglycemic clamp procedure. From "Insulin Action and Secretion in Endurance-Trained and Untrained Humans" by D.S. King, G.P. Dalsky, M.A. Staten, W.E. Clutter, D.R. van Houten, and J.O. Holloszy, 1987, *Journal of Applied Physiology*, **63**, 2247–2252. Reprinted by permission.

immobilization causes rapidly developing insulin resistance of muscle (Seider, Nicholson, & Booth, 1982).

The mechanism behind the training-induced increase in insulin action in muscle seems to be related to increased insulin binding and possibly to increased insulin receptor tyrosine kinase activity at low insulin concentrations (Dohm, Sinha, & Caro, 1987). However, recent findings indicate a close correlation between the activity of lipoprotein lipase in skeletal muscle and muscle insulin sensitivity (Kiens, Lithell, Mikines, & Richter, 1988). Furthermore, it was found that insulin decreased muscle lipoprotein lipase activity, and the decrease correlated closely with the insulin-induced increased muscle glucose uptake (Kiens et al.). The functional meaning of these correlations remains to be elucidated; however, they do suggest that the well-known interrelationship between glucose and lipid metabolism may be more complex than just an effect of circulating free fatty acids on glucose utilization. For instance, one could envision that lipoprotein lipase action on circulating triglycerides locally could increase the concentration of free fatty acids and thereby cause a local decrease in glucose utilization. In this light, the correlation between

Table 1   Glucose Uptake in Control (C) and Immobilized (IM) Thighs

Plasma insulin (μU/ml)	Basal ~9	Insulin I ~65	Insulin II ~440
Glucose uptake (μmol/min)	(C) 40 ± 9	299 ± 60*	644 ± 22*
	(IM) 35 ± 6	224 ± 65	559 ± 18

Note. Values are $M \pm$ SE of 5 subjects. Glucose uptake was measured simultaneously across control and 7-days-immobilized thighs during an euglycemic clamp procedure.

* $p < .05$ compared with IM thigh.

the insulin-induced decrease in lipoprotein lipase activity and the increase in glucose uptake becomes meaningful. However, such a scheme does not explain the apparent association between muscle lipoprotein lipase activity and muscle insulin sensitivity.

Endurance training increases lipoprotein lipase activity in skeletal muscle (Kiens & Lithell, 1985), and the increase in HDL-cholesterol that occurs after endurance training (for references see Lithell, 1986) can be explained at least in part by HDL-cholesterol formation in the trained muscle, possibly related to the training-induced increase in lipoprotein lipase activity (Kiens & Lithell). Because insulin decreases the activity of lipoprotein lipase in muscle, the training-induced decrease in plasma insulin concentrations may be important for the maintenance of high lipoprotein lipase activity in skeletal muscle and thereby for the formation of HDL-cholesterol.

Thus, in the trained state lower insulin concentrations are found. The health benefits of this adaptation may relate to the fact that hyperinsulinemia (possibly due to its effect on lipoprotein lipase in muscle?) has been suggested as an independent risk factor for development of arteriosclerosis (Stern & Haffner, 1986). Thus, training diminishes or abolishes this risk factor.

When Should Studies at Rest Be Carried Out?

Even single bouts of exercise increase muscle insulin sensitivity (Richter, Garetto, Goodman, & Ruderman, 1982), and it appears that a rather large part of the training-induced increase in insulin sensitivity is due to effects of the last training session (Heath et al., 1983; Ivy, Young, McLane, Fell, & Holloszy, 1983). An interesting general question when one considers effects of training is how long after the last exercise session one should study effects of training so as to avoid "acute" effects of the session. The answer is complicated because it could be argued that the "normal" situation for a trained subject, who naturally exercises frequently, is to be in the postexercise period, and as such the subject should be studied the day after the last exercise bout. On the other hand, it has been the custom to study trained subjects 2 to 4 days after the last exercise session, based on evidence that most effects of a single exercise session vanish during such a time span.

Cardiovascular Effects

Cardiovascular effects of exercise training are well known. Some of them could be due to changes in tissue sensitivity to hormones or neurotransmitters or both. For instance, the resting bradycardia found in trained subjects could be due to decreased activity of sympathetic cardiac nerves, to decreased cardiac sensitivity to norepinephrine, or to increased parasympathetic activity. However, in this case it has been convincingly shown that the training-induced resting bradycardia in humans is due not to decreased cardiac sensitivity to catecholamines (Lehmann et al., 1984; Svedenhag, 1985; Williams, Eden, Moll, Lester, & Wallace, 1981) but rather to altered neural activity to the heart, primarily increased parasympathetic activity (Frick, Elovainio, & Somer, 1967).

• Abnormalities in Hypothalamic-Pituitary-Ovarian Function in Endurance-Trained Female Athletes

Extensive endurance training is associated with secondary amenorrhea, that is, the absence of menstrual cycles and low circulating estrogen concentrations in females who previously have had menstrual cycles. The occurrence of athletic amenorrhea seems to be higher in runners (up to 50% in competitive runners) and ballet dancers than in swimmers and bicyclists; the explanation for this is unknown (Loucks & Horvath, 1985). Athletic amenorrhea is characterized by low circulating estrogen concentrations and absence of normal preovulatory increases in follicle-stimulating hormone (FSH) concentrations (Loucks & Horvath) as well as decreased frequency and amplitude of LH pulses (Fisher, Nelson, Frontera, Turksoy, & Evans, 1986). Data suggest that the underlying endocrine disorder is located in the hypothalamus because it has been shown in four women with athletic amenorrhea that the FSH response to gonadotropin-releasing hormone (GnRH) stimulation was normal (McArthur et al., 1980; Wakat, Sweeney, & Rogol, 1982).

The exact cause of athletic amenorrhea is not known. It has been associated with late menarche (M.E. Nelson et al., 1986; Wakat et al.)—possibly training induced?—as well as with psychological stress (Galle, Freeman, Galle, Huggins, & Sondheimer, 1983), but clear evidence is lacking. It has also been proposed that the disorder is associated with low body fat, but recent studies have found the same body fat content in amenorrheic and eumenorrheic subjects (M.E. Nelson et al.; Sanborn, Albrecht, & Wagner, 1987). However, amenorrheic subjects have been found to consume fewer calories than eumenorrheic controls (M.E. Nelson et al.) and, of the amenorrheic runners, 82% consumed less protein than the U.S. dietary allowance (M.E. Nelson et al.). Whether amenorrhea is caused by dietary insufficiency or whether abnormal eating behavior is just another symptom of a disorder that also features amenorrhea is not clear.

In eumenorrheic women the concentrations of estradiol and progesterone increased similarly in trained as well as untrained women during exercise, probably reflecting that decreased clearance was the common factor responsible for the increased hormone concentrations. This was supported by the finding of decreased FSH and LH concentrations during exercise (Keizer, Kuipers, de Haan, Beckers, & Habets, 1987). In a longitudinal study over 3 months, basal estradiol and testosterone concentrations in the luteal phase were decreased after training, and basal ACTH and dehydroepiandrosterone were decreased in both the follicular and luteal phases (Keizer, Kuipers, de Haan, Janssen et al., 1987). Bullen et al. (1985) found menstrual disorders in a majority of previously regularly menstruating women who embarked on a strenuous endurance training program for 2 months.

Amenorrhea is not the only endocrine disorder experienced by female athletes; menstruating female endurance athletes may experience anovulatory cycles characterized by a short luteal phase and abnormally low increases in progesterone and estrogens (Bonen, Belcastro, Ling, & Simpson, 1981). Furthermore, mild thyroidal impairment was found in women who increased their running mileage from 13.5 to 30 miles per week (Boyden, Pamenter, Stanforth, Rotkis, & Wilmore, 1982).

Functional Significance

Athletic amenorrhea is associated with increased incidence of musculoskeletal injuries (Lloyd et al., 1986) and a decreased bone mineral content of the spine (Drinkwater et al., 1984; Fisher et al., 1986; M.E. Nelson et al., 1986). The latter disorder is not explicable by inadequate calcium intake (Drinkwater et al., 1984; M.E. Nelson et al., 1986), but probably is due to decreased circulating estrogen concentrations (Figure 4). It differs from postmenopausal bone loss by affecting primarily weight-bearing bones. Many years of athletic amenorrhea may thus place these women at risk for early postmenopausal osteoporosis. Hormonal replacement therapy with cyclical estrogen treatment may with this background be wise in athletic amenorrhea. On the other hand, such treatment may further suppress the hypothalamic-pituitary-ovarian axis and could therefore lead to a lower rate of reversibility of amenorrhea when training intensity is decreased. However, information is lacking on this subject. It is also of interest to study whether increasing calorie and particularly protein intake may alleviate athletic amenorrhea.

Mechanisms Behind Neuroendocrine Adaptations to Exercise Training

Not much is known about the actual mechanisms eliciting the hormonal adaptations to exercise training. As mentioned earlier, the decrease in

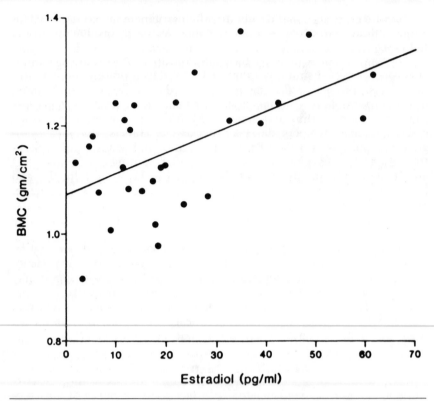

Figure 4. Relationship of bone mineral content (BMC) and serum estradiol levels. Thirty percent of the variation in BMC is explained by the variation in estradiol. From "Bone Mineral Content and Levels of Gonadotropins and Estrogens in Amenorrheic Running Women" by E.C. Fisher, M.E. Nelson, W.R. Frontere, R.N. Turksoy, and W.J. Evans, 1986, *Journal of Clinical Endocrinology and Metabolism,* **62,** 1232–1236. Reprinted by permission.

response of many hormones during exercise occurs rapidly after onset of training and before increases in $\dot{V}O_2$max are expected to occur. Thus, the hormonal response to exercise is not so tightly linked to the relative exercise intensity as most studies suggest. A first question to be asked is whether the hormonal adaptations to training are primary or are elicited secondarily because of changes in target tissue sensitivity. This question is hard to answer unequivocally, but if as an example we consider changes in tissue insulin sensitivity after training, then it seems to be clear that in muscle, contractions per se increase insulin sensitivity independently of hormonal influences (Richter, Ploug, & Galbo, 1985). Thus, because muscle is the largest insulin-sensitive organ in the body it is a necessary consequence for the body to decrease insulin secretion following exercise compared with secretion in the absence of exercise. In this case, then, it might seem reasonable to suggest that changes in hormone secretion are secondary to changes in target tissue sensitivity.

However, tissues that do not directly participate in exercise (such as adipose tissue) may also acquire a higher degree of insulin sensitivity following training (James et al., 1985). Furthermore, the endocrine pancreas adapts to the state of higher insulin sensitivity by acquiring a lower glucose sensitivity (King et al., 1987), and this adaptation apparently takes place within the b-cell, because the adaptation can also be found during in vitro incubations of isolated islets of Langerhans (Galbo, Hedeskov, Capito, & Vinten, 1981). This sequence may not apply to all hormone systems. For instance, in the case of catecholamine secretion during exercise, it is quite unclear which factors can cause a marked reduction in secretion during exercise at a given work load within a week of training.

Another question then is what the mechanism is behind the target tissue adaptation that occurs during training. In the case of muscle adaptation at the level of oxidative enzymes and enzymes in the respiratory chain, it seems clear that muscle contractions per se, devoid even of nervous trophic influence, can cause enzymatic adaptation (Salmons & Henriksson, 1981). As alluded to previously, contraction-induced increases in insulin sensitivity also occur because of contractions per se. The question then arises, How do contractions per se bring about these changes? The answer to this important question is not yet known. We have recently shown (Richter, Cleland, Rattigan, & Clark, 1987) that muscle contractions induce translocation of protein kinase C from the cytosol to the membrane fraction of rat skeletal muscle (Figure 5). Translocation is regarded as activation, because protein kinase C is active only in the presence of phospholipids. Furthermore, diacylglycerol (an activator of protein kinase C) is produced during muscle contractions (S. Rattigan & M. Clark, personal communication). Thus, during muscle contractions, cytosolic calcium increases, protein kinase C is translocated to the membrane fraction, and diacylglycerol is produced.

These events all point to activation of protein kinase C during muscle contractions. Muscle contractions may give rise to long-term translocation of protein kinase C (Alkon & Rasmussen, 1988; Richter et al., 1987), but it is also conceivable that protein kinase C may oscillate from the cytosol to the membrane fraction during each muscle contraction as intracellular calcium concentrations oscillate (Figure 6). The reason for this hypothesis is that in homogenates of hearts (S. Rattigan & M. Clark, personal communication) and of cultured cells (Gopalakrishna, Barsky, Thomas, & Anderson, 1986), the subcellular distribution of protein kinase C is determined by the concentration of calcium in the homogenate: the higher the calcium concentration the higher the activity in the membrane fraction and the lower the activity in the cytosol.

Whereas the physiologically important substrates for protein kinase C in the intact cell are not well known, protein kinase C has been implicated in regulation of growth (for references see Alkon & Rasmussen, 1988), and it is possible that its activation may be involved in training-induced adaptations in muscle. Unraveling the molecular mechanisms involved in training-induced adaptive changes in muscle sensitivity to hormones is a major task for future research.

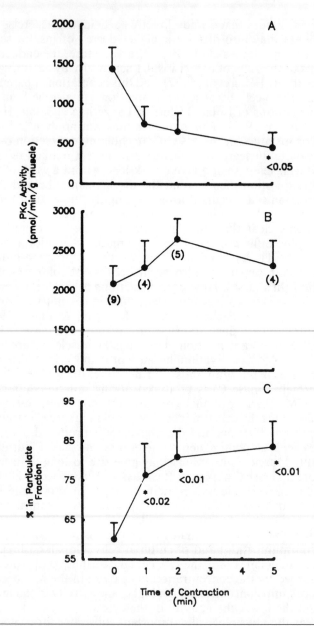

Figure 5. Effect of electrical stimulation-induced contractions of muscle on protein kinase C activity in cytosolic (A) and particulate (B) fractions, and on the percentage of protein kinase C activity in the particulate fraction (C). From "Contraction-Associated Translocation of Protein Kinase C in Rat Skeletal Muscle" by E.A. Richter, P.J.F. Cleland, S. Rattigan, and M.G. Clark, 1987, *FEBS Letters,* **217,** 232–236. Reprinted by permission.

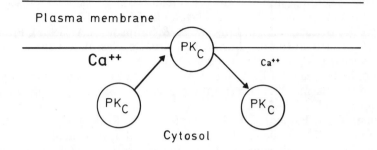

PK$_C$ may oscillate between cytosol and
plasma membrane as intracellular Ca^{++} changes

Figure 6.   Hypothetical oscillation of protein kinase C during muscle contractions. When intracellular calcium concentrations are high (during depolarization), protein kinase C moves to the plasma membrane, and during repolarization the enzyme moves back to the cytosol.

Although it is possible to envision a scenario for adaptations to exercise within the active muscles, it becomes more difficult to understand how adaptations occur in tissues that are not directly involved in exercise, such as adipose tissue and the endocrine pancreas. These adaptations may occur as a consequence of repeated bursts of sympathetic nervous activity elicited during exercise, but definitive studies are lacking.

Another important question is this: What is the mechanism behind training-induced amenorrhea? This disorder seems to be due to changes in the hypothalamus or areas of the brain above the hypothalamus, because the pituitary and ovarian response to LH-releasing hormone seem to be normal. Aside from theoretical interest this question also has large practical implications for the not-so-few female athletes affected by this potentially troublesome condition.

Acknowledgments

Cited studies by the author were supported by grants from the Danish Medical Research Council, NOVO Research Foundation, the Danish Sports Research Council, P. Carl Petersens Foundation, Nordisk Insulin Foundation, and the Danish Diabetes Association.

References

Alkon, D.L., & Rasmussen, H. (1988). A spacial-temporal model of cell activation. *Science, 239*, 998-1004.

Berger, M., Kemmer, F.W., Becker, K., Herberg, L., Schwener, M., Gjinavci, A., & Berchtold, P. (1979). Effect of physical training on glucose tolerance and on glucose metabolism of skeletal muscle in anesthetised normal rats. *Diabetologia,* **16,** 179–184.

Bonen, A., Belcastro, A.N., Ling, W.Y., & Simpson, A.A. (1981). Profiles of selected hormones during menstrual cycles of teenage athletes. *Journal of Applied Physiology,* **50,** 545–551.

Buono, M.J., Yeager, J.E., & Sucec, A.A. (1987). Effect of aerobic training on the plasma ACTH response to exercise. *Journal of Applied Physiology,* **63,** 2499–2501.

Boyden, T.W., Pamenter, R.W., Stanforth, P., Rotkis, T., & Wilmore, J.H. (1982). Evidence for mild thyroidal impairment in women undergoing endurance training. *Journal of Clinical Endocrinology and Metabolism,* **53,** 53–56.

Bukowiecki, L., Lupien, J., Follea, N., Paradis, A., Richard, D., & Le Blanc, J. (1980). Mechanism of enhanced lipolysis in adipose tissue of exercise-trained rats. *American Journal of Physiology,* **239,** E422–E429.

Bullen, B.A., Skrinar, G.S., Beitins, I.Z., von Mering, G., Turnbull, B.A., & McArthur, J.W. (1985). Induction of menstrual disorders by strenuous exercise in untrained women. *New England Journal of Medicine,* **312,** 1349–1353.

Craig, B.W., Hammons, G.T., Garthwaite, S.M., Jarett, L., & Holloszy, J.O. (1981). Adaptation of fat cells to exercise: Response of glucose uptake and oxidation to insulin. *Journal of Applied Physiology,* **51,** 1500–1506.

Crampes, F., Beauville, M., Riviere, D., & Garrigues, M. (1986). Effect of physical training in humans on the response of isolated fat cells to epinephrine. *Journal of Applied Physiology,* **61,** 25–29.

Dohm, G.L., Sinha, M.K., & Caro, J.F. (1987). Insulin receptor binding and protein kinase activity in muscles of trained rats. *American Journal of Physiology,* **252,** E170–E175.

Drinkwater, B.L., Nilson, K., Chestnut, C.H., Bremner, W.J., Shainholtz, S., & Southworth, M.B. (1984). Bone mineral content of amenorrheic and eumenorrheic athletes. *New England Journal of Medicine,* **311,** 277–281.

Fisher, E.C., Nelson, M.E., Frontera, W.R., Turksoy, R.N., & Evans, W.J. (1986). Bone mineral content and levels of gonadotropins and estrogens in amenorrheic running women. *Journal of Clinical Endocrinology and Metabolism,* **62,** 1232–1236.

Fitzgerald, W. (1981). Labile hypertension and jogging: New diagnostic tool or spurious discovery? *British Medical Journal,* **282,** 542–544.

Frick, M.H., Elovainio, R.O., & Somer, T. (1967). The mechanism of bradycardia evoked by physical training. *Cardiologia,* **51,** 46–54.

Galbo, H. (1986). Autonomic neuroendocrine responses to exercise. *Scandinavian Journal of Sports Sciences,* **8,** 3–17.

Galbo, H., Hedeskov, C.S., Capito, K., & Vinten, S. (1981). The effect of physical training on insulin secretion of rat pancreatic islets. *Acta Physiologica Scandinavica,* **111,** 75–79.

Galle, P.C., Freeman, E.W., Galle, M.G., Huggins, G.R., & Sondheimer, S.J. (1983). Physiologic and psychologic profiles in a survey of women runners. *Fertility and Sterility,* **39,** 633–639.

Gopalakrishna, R., Barsky, S.H., Thomas, T.P., & Anderson, W.B. (1986). Factors influencing chelator-stable, detergent-extractable, phorbol diester-induced membrane association of protein kinase C. *Journal of Biological Chemistry,* **261,** 16438–16445.

Hackney, A.C., Sinning, W.E., & Bruot, B.C. (1988). Reproductive hormonal profiles of endurance-trained and untrained males. *Medicine and Science in Sports and Exercise,* **20,** 60–65.

Hartley, L.H., Mason, J.W., Hogan, R.P., Jones, L.G., Kotchen, T.A., Mougey, E.H., Wherry, F.E., Pennington, L.L., & Ricketts, P.T. (1972). Multiple hormonal responses to prolonged exercise in relation to physical training. *Journal of Applied Physiology,* **33,** 607–610.

Heath, G.W., Gavin, J.R., III., Hinderliter, J.M., Hagberg, J.M., Bloomfield, S.A., & Holloszy, J.O. (1983). Effects of exercise and lack of exercise on glucose tolerance and insulin sensitivity. *Journal of Applied Physiology,* **55,** 512–517.

Ivy, J.L., Young, J.C., McLane, J.A., Fell, R.D., & Holloszy, J.O. (1983). Exercise training and glucose uptake by skeletal muscle in rats. *Journal of Applied Physiology,* **55,** 1393–1396.

James, D.E., Kraegen, E.W., & Chisholm, D.J. (1985). Effects of exercise training on in vivo insulin action in individual tissues of the rat. *Journal of Clinical Investigation,* **76,** 657–666.

Jennings, G., Nelson, L., Nestel, P., Esler, M., Korner, P., Burton, D., & Bazelmans, J. (1986). The effects of changes in physical activity on major cardiovascular risk factors, hemodynamics, sympathetic function, and glucose utilization in man: A controlled study of four levels of activity. *Circulation,* **73,** 30–40.

Keizer, H.A., Kuipers, H., de Haan, J., Janssen, G.M.E., Beckers, E., Habets, L., van Kranenburg, G., & Geurten, P. (1987). Effect of a 3-month endurance training program on metabolic and multiple hormonal responses to exercise. *International Journal of Sports Medicine,* **8,** 154–160.

Keizer, H.A., Kuipers, H., de Haan, J., Beckers, E., & Habets, L. (1987). Multiple hormonal responses to physical exercise in eumenorrheic trained and untrained women. *International Journal of Sports Medicine,* **8,** 139–150.

Kiens, B., & Lithell, H. (1985). Lipoprotein metabolism related to adaptations in human skeletal muscle (abstract). *Clinical Science,* **5,** (Suppl. 4), 108.

Kiens, B., Lithell, H., Mikines, K.J., & Richter, E.A. (1988). Muscle-LPLA is decreased by glucose and insulin (abstract). *Medicine and Science in Sports and Exercise* **20** (Suppl.), 573.

King, D.S., Dalsky, G.P., Staten, M.A., Clutter, W.E., van Houten, D.R., & Holloszy, J.O. (1987). Insulin action and secretion in endurance-trained and untrained humans. *Journal of Applied Physiology,* **63,** 2247–2252.

Kjær, M., Christensen, N.J., Sonne, B., Richter, E.A., & Galbo, H. (1985). Effect of exercise on epinephrine turnover in trained and untrained male subjects. *Journal of Applied Physiology,* **59,** 1061–1067.

Kjær, M., Farrell, P.A., Christensen, N.J., & Galbo, H. (1986). Increased epinephrine response and inaccurate glucoregulation in exercising athletes. *Journal of Applied Physiology,* **61,** 1693–1700.

Kjær, M., & Galbo, H. (1988). Effect of physical training on the capacity to secrete epinephrine. *Journal of Applied Physiology,* **64,** 11–16.

Kjær, M., Mikines, K.J., Christensen, N.J., Tronier, B., Vinten, J., Sonne, B., Richter, E.A., & Galbo, H. (1984). Glucose turnover and hormonal changes during insulin-induced hypoglycemia in trained humans. *Journal of Applied Physiology,* **57,** 21–27.

Koivisto, V., Hendler, R., Nadel, E., & Felig, P. (1982). Influence of physical training on the fuel-hormone response to prolonged low intensity exercise. *Metabolism,* **31,** 192–196.

Kuoppasalmi, K., Näveri, H., Kosunen, K., Härkönen, M., & Adlercreutz, H. (1981). Plasma steroid levels in muscular exercise. In J. Poortmans and G. Niset (Eds.), *Biochemistry of exercise, IV-B,* pp. 149–160. Baltimore: University Park Press.

Lehmann, M., Dickhuth, H.H., Schmid, P., Porzig, H., & Keul, J. (1984). Plasma catecholamines, beta-adrenergic receptors, and isoproterenol sensitivity in endurance trained and non-endurance trained volunteers. *European Journal of Applied Physiology,* **52,** 362–369.

Lithell, H.O. (1986). Lipoprotein metabolism and physical training in normal man and diabetic and cardiac patients. In B. Saltin (Ed.), *Biochemistry of Exercise VI, Vol. 16,* pp. 279–309. Champaign, IL: Human Kinetics.

Lloyd, T., Triantafyllou, S.J., Baker, E.R., Houts, P.S., Whiteside, J.A., Kalenak, A., & Stumpf, P.G. (1986). Women athletes with menstrual irregularity have increased musculoskeletal injuries. *Medicine and Science in Sports and Exercise,* **18,** 374–379.

Lohmann, D., Liebold, G., Heilmann, W., Senger, H., & Pohl, A. (1978). Diminished insulin response in highly trained athletes. *Metabolism,* **27,** 521–524.

Loucks, A.B., & Horvath, S.M. (1985). Athletic amenorrhea: A review. *Medicine and Science in Sports and Exercise,* **17,** 56–72.

Luger, A., Deuster, P.A., Kyle, S.B., Gallucci, W.T., Montgomery, L.C., Gold, P.W., Loriaux, D.L., & Chrousos, G.P. (1987). Acute hypothalamic-pituitary-adrenal responses to the stress of treadmill exercise. *New England Journal of Medicine,* **316,** 1309–1315.

McArthur, J.W., Bullen, B.A., Beitins, I.Z., Pagano, M., Badger, T.M., & Klibanski, A. (1980). Hypothalamic amenorrhea in runners of normal body composition. *Endocrine Research Communications,* **7,** 13–25.

Mikines, K.J., Dela, F., Sonne, B., Farrell, P.A., Richter, E.A., & Galbo, H. (1987). Insulin action and secretion in man: Effects of different levels of physical activity. *Canadian Journal of Sports Sciences,* **12**(Suppl. 1), 113–116.

Mitchell, J.H., Kaufman, M.P., & Iwamoto, G.A. (1983). The exercise pressor reflex: Its cardiovascular effects, afferent mechanisms and central pathways. *Annual Review of Physiology, 45,* 229–242.

Mondon, C.E., Dolkas, C.B., & Reaven, G.M. (1980). Site of enhanced insulin sensitivity in exercise-trained rats at rest. *American Journal of Physiology, 239,* E169–E177.

Nelson, L., Jennings, G.L., Esler, M.D., & Korner, P.I. (1986). Effect of changing levels of physical activity on blood-pressure and haemodynamics in essential hypertension. *Lancet, 2,* 473–476.

Nelson, M.E., Fisher, E.C., Catsos, P.D., Meredith, C.N., Turksoy, R.N., & Evans, W.J. (1986). Diet and bone status in amenorrheic runners. *American Journal of Clinical Nutrition, 43,* 910–916.

Richter, E.A., Christensen, N.J., Ploug, T., & Galbo, H. (1984). Endurance training augments the stimulatory effect of epinephrine on oxygen consumption in perfused skeletal muscle. *Acta Physiologica Scandinavica, 120,* 613–615.

Richter, E.A., Cleland, P.J.F., Rattigan, S., & Clark, M.G. (1987). Contraction-associated translocation of protein kinase C in rat skeletal muscle. *FEBS Letters, 217,* 232–236.

Richter, E.A., Garetto, L.P., Goodman, M.N., & Ruderman, N.B. (1982). Muscle glucose metabolism following exercise in the rat. *Journal of Clinical Investigation, 69,* 785–793.

Richter, E.A., Kjær, M., & Galbo, H. (1986). Endurance training does not increase muscle glycogenolysis, ' AMP production and phosphorylase activation in response to epinephrine. *Acta Physiologica Scandinavica, 126,* 26A.

Richter, E.A., Ploug, T., & Galbo, H. (1985). Increased muscle glucose uptake after exercise. *Diabetes, 34,* 1041–1048.

Richter, E.A., Ruderman, N.B., & Galbo, H. (1982). Alpha and beta adrenergic effects of metabolism in contracting, perfused muscle. *Acta Physiologica Scandinavica, 116,* 215–222.

Rodnick, K.J., Haskell, W.L., Swislocki, A.L.M., Foley, J.E., & Reaven, G.M. (1987). Improved insulin action in muscle, liver and adipose tissue in physically trained human subjects. *American Journal of Physiology, 253,* E489–E495.

Salmons, S., & Henriksson, J. (1981). The adaptive response of skeletal muscle to increased use. *Muscle and Nerve, 4,* 94–105.

Sanborn, C.F., Albrecht, B.H., & Wagner, W.W. (1987). Athletic amenorrhea: Lack of association with body fat. *Medicine and Science in Sports and Exercise, 19,* 207–212.

Savard, G., Strange, S., Kiens, B., Richter, E.A., Christensen, N.J., & Saltin, B. (1987). Noradrenaline spillover during exercise in active versus resting skeletal muscle in man. *Acta Physiologica Scandinavica, 131,* 507–515.

Seals, D.R., & Hagberg, J.M. (1984). The effect of exercise training on human hypertension: A review. *Medicine and Science in Sports and Exercise, 16,* 207–215.

Seider, M.J., Nicholson, W.F., & Booth, F.W. (1982). Insulin resistance for glucose metabolism in disused soleus muscle of mice. *American Journal of Physiology, 7,* E12–E18.

Stern, M.P., & Haffner, S.M. (1986). Body fat distribution and hyperinsulineamia as risk factors for diabetes and cardiovascular disease. *Arteriosclerosis, 6,* 123–130.

Svedenhag, J. (1985). The sympatho-adrenal system in physical conditioning. *Acta Physiologica Scandinavica, 125*(Suppl. 543), 1–73.

Svedenhag, J., Wallin, B.G., Sundlöf, G., & Henriksson, J. (1984). Skeletal muscle sympathetic activity at rest in trained and untrained subjects. *Acta Physiologica Scandinavica, 120,* 499–504.

Vinten, J., & Galbo, H. (1983). Effect of physical training on transport and metabolism of glucose in adipocytes. *American Journal of Physiology, 244,* E129–E134.

Wakat, D.K., Sweeney, K.A., & Rogol, A.D. (1982). Reproductive system function in women cross-country runners. *Medicine and Science in Sports and Exercise, 14,* 263–269.

Wallin, B.G., Sundlöf, G., Eriksson, B-M., Dominiak, P., Grobecker, H., & Lindblad, L.E. (1981). Plasma noradrenaline correlates to sympathetic muscle nerve activity in normotensive man. *Acta Physiologica Scandinavica, 111,* 69–73.

Wilcox, R.G., Bennett, T., Brown, A.M., & MacDonald, I.A. (1982). Is exercise good for high blood pressure? *British Medical Journal, 285,* 767–769.

Williams, R.S., & Bishop, T. (1982). Enhanced receptor-cyclase coupling and augmented catecholamine-stimulated lipolysis in exercising rats. *American Journal of Physiology, 243,* E345–E351.

Williams, R.S., Caron, M.G., and Daniel, K. (1984). Skeletal muscle ß-adrenergic receptors: Variations due to fiber type and training. *American Journal of Physiology, 246,* E160–E167.

Williams, R.S., Eden, R.S., Moll, M.E., Lester, R.M. & Wallace, A.G. (1981). Autonomic mechanisms of training bradycardia: ß-adrenergic receptors in humans. *Journal of Applied Physiology, 51,* 1232–1237.

Winder, W.W., Hagberg, J.M., Hickson, R.C., Ehsani, A.A., & McLane, J.A. (1978). Time course of sympathoadrenal adaptation to endurance exercise training in man. *Journal of Applied Physiology, 45,* 370–374.

Winder, W.W., Hickson, R.C., Hagberg, J.M., Ehsani, A.A., & McLane, J.A. (1979). Training-induced changes in hormonal and metabolic responses to submaximal exercise. *Journal of Applied Physiology, 46,* 766–771.

Wirth, A., Diehm, C., Mayer, H., Mörl, H., Vogel, I., Björntorp, P., & Schlierf, G. (1981). Plasma C-peptide and insulin in trained and untrained subjects. *Journal of Applied Physiology, 50,* 71–77.

Effects of Habitual Exercise on Lipoprotein Metabolism

Peter D. Wood

Stanford Center for Research in Disease Prevention
Palo Alto, California

Several prospective studies, notably those of Paffenbarger, Hyde, Wing, and Steinmetz (1984) in the U.S. and Morris, Everitt, Pollard, and Chave (1980) in England, have provided persuasive, but by no means conclusive, evidence in favor of the contention that regular physical activity, especially in leisure time sports play, continued throughout adult life substantially reduces the incidence of coronary heart disease (CHD). There is some evidence that stroke rates may also be reduced in active people (Paffenbarger et al., 1984). A large, controlled, randomized trial in young, asymptomatic men and women would be required to test the hypothesis rigorously. The costs and ethical problems involved in such a study mean that it will probably never be attempted. We shall be obliged to base public health recommendations in the exercise area on a mass of less-than-conclusive evidence, most of which points in the same direction, as we have done in the area of smoking and health.

Mechanisms proposed for the apparently protective effect of regular exercise include

- improved cardiopulmonary function,
- increased fibrinolytic activity,
- beneficial effects on the behavior of platelets,
- decreased blood pressure levels,
- increased coronary artery bore, and
- salutary effects on the concentrations of serum lipoproteins and apolipoproteins related to risk of CHD and perhaps of stroke.

This brief discussion will focus on the last of these exercise effects.

Cross-Sectional Studies

Risk factors for heart and vascular diseases often flock together: Very active people in our society today tend to be nonsmokers of higher socioeconomic status, for instance. Generally, it seems clear that the effects of increased muscular contraction on plasma lipoproteins are independent of these frequently associated factors. But there are associations so close that the components are only gradually being dissected apart. Regular exercisers tend to be lean, and a training program in sedentary individuals very often leads to loss of body fat. In addition, and paradoxically to some, increased energy expenditure with loss of body fat is often accompanied by *increased* caloric intake (Wood, Terry, & Haskell, 1985). Thus, in the real world, the effects of habitual exercise on lipoprotein metabolism encompass the effects of relatively low body fat content and of relatively high caloric intake (in comparison with sedentary individuals) on lipoprotein metabolism. From a public health viewpoint, increased exercise, decreased body fat, and increased caloric intake should probably be regarded as a "package" that will result from successful attempts to increase physical activity in a community or at a work site.

Numerous cross-sectional studies comparing serum lipoprotein status in groups of relatively active men and women and in groups of relatively sedentary, matched control subjects have been carried out. The consensus is clear (Wood, Williams, & Haskell, 1984) that regularly active runners, cross-country skiers, soccer players, swimmers, and brisk walkers, among other groups studied, tend to have the following characteristics:

- higher serum concentrations of high-density lipoprotein (HDL) cholesterol and total mass, especially the apparently "protective" HDL_2 subfraction;
- lower concentrations of triglycerides and of very low-density lipoprotein (VLDL) cholesterol;
- higher levels of apolipoprotein A-I (the predominant peptide of HDL), which has been shown to be negatively related to risk of CHD;
- good (i.e., "protective") ratios for the serum concentrations of total cholesterol/HDL-cholesterol and of low-density lipoprotein (LDL) cholesterol/HDL-cholesterol.

Most cross-sectional studies have failed to show significantly lower serum levels of total cholesterol or of the atherogenic LDL-cholesterol (Wood et al., 1984). It is of interest that LDL-cholesterol levels are lower in the active groups in a few studies where very dedicated exercisers (for instance, marathon runners) have been compared to sedentary controls (Williams et al., 1986). This is illustrated in Table 1, which also indicates that important changes in the LDL subfractions may occur with exercise that are less apparent from measurements of LDL-cholesterol alone. Reciprocal relationships between serum concentrations of HDL_2 ($F_{1.20}$ 2.0– 9.0) and "small" LDL (S_f 0–7) are seen in comparisons of the active and the sedentary and in longitudinal training studies in which the sedentary become active (Krauss, Williams, Lindgren, & Wood, 1988). The CHD protection associated with high serum levels of HDL_2 might therefore be due to accompanying low levels of "small LDL," since the latter state has recently been shown to characterize individuals with low risk of CHD.

This reciprocal relationship is seen in Table 1, comparing male long-distance runners with sedentary controls of similar age (Williams et al., 1986).

In considering cross-sectional studies it is of interest to remember that very active individuals often have substantially increased plasma volumes compared to sedentary controls. The total circulating mass of HDL in exercisers, with higher plasma HDL concentrations, can therefore be considerably greater than in sedentary individuals. However, it seems probable that the influences of both LDL and HDL on the atherosclerotic process are best expressed in terms of their serum concentrations.

Longitudinal Studies

A number of longitudinal or exercise training studies have been conducted in which sedentary individuals are followed as attempts are made to increase their physical activity levels, for instance in a jogging or walking program. Such studies are not easy to conduct and have often suffered from such deficiencies as inadequate participant numbers; lack of a control group, or of random assignment to exercising or to remaining sedentary; inadequate length of training program; and inappropriate statistical evaluation of data obtained (Wood et al., 1984).

The results of such studies with respect to elevation of HDL-cholesterol level have been considered conflicting, although virtually all training programs of 12 weeks or longer have reported increased HDL-cholesterol levels in the exercising group (the increases frequently being statistically insignificant). Inability to produce a substantial increase in physical activity or fitness in a considerable proportion of the participants, especially in brief studies, undoubtedly has contributed to many negative results. It is certainly unreasonable to expect to mimic the striking fitness differences seen, for instance, in a comparison of marathon runners and sedentary controls, during a training study lasting only a few weeks, even though fitness (measured by maximal oxygen consumption or $\dot{V}O_2$max) may be slightly but significantly increased in that time period. Training studies, when randomized, minimize the problem of self-selection that characterizes cross-sectional studies. In most training studies a significant correlation has been found between the magnitude of the serum HDL-cholesterol increase observed and the amount of exercise performed by the participants, supporting the idea of cause and effect (Wood et al., 1984).

Exercise, Adiposity, and Lipoproteins

Attempts have been made to adjust for adiposity in cross-sectional studies and to hold body weight constant in training studies. There is some indication that exercise level and adiposity level are independent and additive influences on serum HDL-cholesterol (Sopko et al., 1985). However, in a recent study in men, body fat loss by caloric restriction (dieting)

Table 1 Comparison of Age, Body Mass Index, Lipids, Lipoproteins, and Lipoprotein and Hepatic Lipase Measurements in Cross-Sectional Samples of Long-Distance Runners and Sedentary Men[a]

	Runners ($M \pm SD$)	Nonrunners ($M \pm SD$)	Difference ($M \pm SE$)	Significance (P)
Age (yr)	46.9 ± 7.5	45.7 ± 6.1	1.3 ± 2.3	0.81
Body mass index (kg/cm^2)	22.6 ± 2.0	25.1 ± 3.3	−2.5 ± 0.7	0.006
Lipids and lipoproteins				
Plasma total cholesterol (mg/dl)	190.9 ± 36.6	217.0 ± 31.1	−26.1 ± 11.3	0.02
Plasma total triglycerides (mg/dl)	70.8 ± 35.0	123.0 ± 59.3	−52.2 ± 12.5	0.001
Plasma HDL-cholesterol (mg/dl)	64.9 ± 12.5	49.6 ± 8.7	15.3 ± 3.8	0.0001
Serum HDL-mass of $F_{1.20}$0–1.5 (mg/dl)	70.0 ± 13.7	82.3 ± 17.5	−12.3 ± 4.5	0.02
Serum HDL-mass of $F_{1.20}$1.5–2.0 (mg/dl)	51.2 ± 8.4	52.3 ± 7.8	−1.1 ± 2.6	0.98
Serum HDL-mass of $F_{1.20}$2.0–9.0 (mg/dl)	213.0 ± 45.6	144.8 ± 47.9	68.2 ± 14.5	0.0002
Plasma LDL-cholesterol (mg/dl)	116.1 ± 30.7	147.0 ± 27.5	−30.9 ± 9.5	0.004
Serum LDL-mass of S_f0–7 (mg/dl)	138.4 ± 45.3	227.6 ± 67.9	−89.2 ± 15.6	0.0001
Serum LDL-mass of S_f7–12 (mg/dl)	136.7 ± 39.8	134.2 ± 43.8	2.5 ± 12.7	0.85
Serum LDL-mass of S_f12–20 (mg/dl)	34.3 ± 18.2	43.8 ± 20.7	−9.5 ± 5.9	0.16
Plasma VLDL-cholesterol (mg/dl)	9.1 ± 8.3	20.4 ± 11.7	−11.3 ± 2.8	0.001
Serum VLDL-mass of S_f20–400 (mg/dl)	36.8 ± 41.6	106.1 ± 72.0	−69.3 ± 15.0	0.001
Postheparin lipase activity				
Lipoprotein lipase (mEq fatty acid/ml/h)	5.0 ± 1.8	3.6 ± 1/2	1.4 ± 0.6	0.04
Hepatic lipase (mEq fatty acid/ml/h)	4.1 ± 2.1	6.5 ± 2.6	−2.4 ± 0.9	0.02

[a]From Williams et al., 1986. Sample sizes are 12 runners and 64 nonrunners for all lipid and lipoprotein variables, age and body mass index; and 12 runners and 16 nonrunners for lipoprotein and hepatic lipase measurements. All significance levels are obtained from two sample Wilcoxon sign rank tests.

without increased exercise was shown to be about equivalent to similar body fat loss by exercising *without* dieting, with respect to beneficial changes in serum lipoproteins (Wood, Haskell, & Fortmann, 1986). Careful studies and precise thinking are required to elucidate the separate influences of muscular contraction, adiposity, and caloric intake upon serum lipoprotein concentrations in humans. Indeed, in considering adiposity, it is becoming increasingly apparent that the distribution of body fat (for instance, predominantly abdominal versus hip and thigh obesity) is an important factor in relation to lipoprotein pattern (Terry, Stefanick, Krauss, Haskell, & Wood, 1985). And in considering caloric intake, we should recall that several prospective studies have shown that reported caloric intake is a predictor of future CHD, in the sense that higher caloric intakes predict *lower* CHD risk (Gordon et al., 1981).

Mechanisms

The metabolic changes underlying the serum lipoprotein concentration changes produced by increased exercise are not fully understood. The activities of two key enzymes—lipoprotein lipase and hepatic lipase—are associated cross-sectionally with physical activity level and change with increased endurance exercise. Lipoprotein lipase, which has a major role in conversion of very low-density lipoprotein (VLDL) to HDL, is more active in runners than in sedentary people and is increased by exercise. Hepatic lipase, which appears to play a major role in the conversion of HDL_2 to HDL_3 and participates in the conversion of VLDL, intermediate density lipoprotein, and large LDL to "small" LDL, is *less* active in exercisers and is *decreased* by increased exercise (Stefanick, Terry, Haskell, & Wood, 1988). These changes in enzyme activity with exercise are correlated with changes in the serum lipoprotein profile (Stefanick et al.).

Increases in lipoprotein lipase activity in cardiac and skeletal muscle with exercise are specifically associated with increased muscular activity. Lipoprotein lipase activity is elevated in working versus resting muscle, and this is associated with increases in HDL and HDL_2 concentrations in the venous blood of the working muscle, relative to its arterial blood. Lipoprotein lipase activity (determined in serum following heparin infusion) has been shown to be positively correlated with $\dot{V}O_2$max (Stefanick et al., 1988).

Decreases in hepatic lipase activity post-heparin and the associated increases in HDL and HDL_2 are strongly associated with weight loss, at least in moderately overweight men who take up an exercise program (Stefanick et al., 1988). Decreased body fat may be one of the most important metabolic consequences of a training program, leading to decreased hepatic lipase activity and so to increased serum HDL and HDL_2 levels. Hepatic lipase activity seems to have a strong genetic component, which may underlie reported genetic regulation of serum HDL concentration and HDL subfraction distribution.

Exercise may also influence lipoprotein concentrations through selective effects on the distribution and lipolytic activity of adipose tissue.

Adipocytes in the abdominal region are more responsive to catechol-amine-induced lipolysis than femoral adipocytes. Selective loss of ab-dominal fat, versus femoral and gluteal fat, induced by exercise, would decrease waist-to-hip ratio, which in turn has been shown to correlate strongly with plasma HDL-cholesterol and HDL_2-mass concentration (Terry et al., 1985) and with risk of CHD death (Lapidus et al., 1984). Changes in lipoprotein metabolism resulting from increased exercise level may therefore result in part from an overall change in adipocyte adre-nergic sensitivity or a redistribution of body fat within regions of different adipocyte sensitivity; or, both mechanisms may operate simultaneously. This is an area of considerable interest with respect to further research, because it relates importantly to both exercise and weight control in relation to CHD risk.

Important determinants of serum LDL-cholesterol concentration are the number and turnover of LDL-receptors in the liver. Because very active individuals tend to have lower serum levels of LDL-cholesterol (as illustrated in Table 1), it would seem of considerable interest to in-vestigate LDL-receptor activity in the livers of very active versus seden-tary individuals. This is clearly a difficult study to carry out in humans, and apparently no data are available. Animal studies may shed some light on this interesting area.

Exercise and Coronary Heart Disease

It is now generally accepted that increased exercise, frequently with ac-companying loss of body fat, does result in changes in serum lipoproteins and apolipoproteins that predict reduced risk of CHD. This seems to be true for men and women, old and young. It should be noted that the most noticeable effect of exercise on serum lipoproteins—an elevation of HDL-cholesterol—has not been shown entirely convincingly in a con-trolled trial to reduce risk of CHD, whereas lowering LDL-cholesterol has been shown clearly to confer benefit. Although a trial specifically designed to test the hypothesis that raising serum HDL-cholesterol level in high-risk individuals reduces incidence of CHD and stroke has not been conducted to date, analysis of the results of the Lipid Research Clinics Coronary Primary Prevention Trial (1984) and the Helsinki Heart Study (Frick et al., 1987) lend strong support to the idea. The former trial used the drug cholestyramine, which primarily lowers serum LDL-cholesterol but secondarily elevates HDL-cholesterol modestly. Analysis of data from this trial suggests that lipoprotein change contributes in-dependently to reduction of CHD risk and that the effect is related to the degree of increase in HDL-cholesterol concentration. The Helsinki trial, using the drug gemfibrozil, produced a pronounced effect on serum HDL-cholesterol (elevated) and a slightly less pronounced effect on LDL-cholesterol plus VLDL-cholesterol (lowered). Preliminary analyses of re-sults from this trial strongly suggest that HDL-cholesterol elevation has a "protective" effect in relation to CHD (Frick et al.).

Public Health Issues

There is currently great enthusiasm for reducing the nation's risk of developing coronary heart disease by improving serum lipoprotein status, most importantly lowering serum LDL-cholesterol levels and elevating HDL-cholesterol levels, in many American adults (Consensus Development Panel, 1985). In view of the pronounced salutary effects of increased exercise level, with concomitant reduction of adiposity, upon the LDL/HDL ratio of serum, it is my opinion that exercise has been relatively neglected as an important hygienic approach to the problem (National Cholesterol Education Program, 1987). Dietary change will no doubt remain the primary approach to LDL-cholesterol reduction, but the adoption of an exercise program is clearly a desirable additional recommendation for many sedentary people.

Of particular concern is the possibility that new "miracle" drugs, such as the HMG CoA reductase inhibitor lovastatin, may be used prematurely in many individuals with only moderate elevations of LDL-cholesterol without an adequate trial of increased exercise and decreased body weight. This is particularly worrying because so much of our population is "relatively sedentary and moderately overweight." Premature administration of such drugs, often with intention to treat for life, exposes this large group of citizens to the drugs' possibly detrimental long-term effects and deprives them of the health benefits resulting from increased fitness and decreased adiposity. The undeniable "ease of administration" of the new drugs (one to four pills a day, with few immediately obvious side effects) should not relieve us of the responsibility to promote important lifestyle changes.

Very small or infrequent amounts of exercise have little effect on risk, as assessed by changes in serum lipoprotein levels: "Easy does it" does *not* "do it all," as has been claimed by some in the popular press recently. There is probably an approximately linear response between low and quite-high levels of physical activity, which is consistent with the observations of Paffenbarger et al. (1984) of reduced risk of CHD in Harvard alumni with increasing levels of habitual leisure time activity. It seems probable that the popular, accessible, and relatively safe activity of brisk walking is a very valuable way to control weight and improve serum lipoprotein status. This will be no less true if it is established that more vigorous forms of exercise are even better in these respects, as seems probable.

Future Investigations

Physical activity and weight control have suffered Cinderella status as research areas for many years, so that much remains to be done to improve our knowledge of these enormously important topics, both from basic science and public health viewpoints. The investigations will require carefully controlled clinical research unit conditions in some cases, and, where there is true need, animal studies in others. But probably the greatest need is for studies in moderately large groups of free-living individuals in real-life situations, studies which are at the same time well-designed and scientifically sound.

Some of the more urgent research areas are these:

- With respect to effects of exercise on serum lipoproteins, how much exercise is enough? Is brisk walking adequate? How frequently should exercise be performed? How intensely?
- Can the frequently concomitant physiological changes—increased physical activity and decreased body fat content—be further differentiated with respect to their influences on lipoprotein metabolism? How important is fat loss from specific regions or redistribution of body fat with exercise?
- The interaction of insulin, catecholamines, and hepatic and lipoprotein lipase and their influence on lipoprotein metabolism needs further study, particularly in humans. The effects of increased exercise and decreased body fat on these interactions is of great interest.
- The effect of exercise, particularly in humans, upon the number and turnover of LDL receptors in the liver and other tissues is an exciting and important research area.
- Finally, there is great need for behavioral studies directed at better understanding what factors motivate people to exercise and how these might be modified. An improved mechanism for directing people toward types of exercise that they will stay with happily for most of their lives is particularly needed.

Summary

In summary, habitual exercise in men and women, old and young, is associated with putatively beneficial serum lipoprotein concentrations, and adoption of an aerobic exercise program by sedentary people leads to improved lipoprotein status with respect to CHD risk. Work is urgently needed to improve our knowledge of the influence on lipoproteins of type, intensity, duration, and frequency of exercise, so that public health messages can be made more specific. Increased exercise level is usually accompanied by decreased adiposity and increased caloric intake, and these concomitant changes probably contribute to the overall effect on lipoprotein metabolism of a physically active lifestyle. Further work is required to elucidate the relative influences of muscular contraction, loss of body fat, and increased caloric intake, considered separately, on lipoprotein concentrations. The mechanism or mechanisms by which increased exercise levels change lipoprotein levels and lipoprotein metabolism are not entirely clear, and this area needs further study. However, it seems very probable that changes in the activity of lipoprotein lipase and hepatic lipase contribute importantly to these mechanisms. Behavioral investigations designed to increase lifelong participation in appropriate endurance exercise are also urgently needed.

References

Consensus Development Panel. (1985). Lowering blood cholesterol to prevent heart disease. *Journal of the American Medical Association,* **253,** 2080–2086.

Frick, M.H., Elo, O., Haapa, K., Heinonen, O.P., Heinsalmi, P., Helo, P., Huttanen, J.K., Kaiteniemi, P., Koskinen, P., Manninen, V., Maenpaa, H., Malkonen, M., Manttari, M., Norola, S., Pasternack, A., Pikkarainen, J., Romo, M., Sjoblom, R., & Nikkila, E.A. (1987). Helsinki Heart Study: Primary-prevention trial with gemfibrozil in middle-aged men with dyslipidemia. *New England Journal of Medicine,* **317,** 1237–1245.

Gordon, T., Kagen, A., Garcia-Palmieri, M., Kannel, W.B., Zukel, W.J., Tillotson, J., Sorlie, P., & Hjortland, M. (1981). Diet and its relationship to coronary heart disease and death in three populations. *Circulation,* **63,** 500–515.

Krauss, R.M., Williams, P.T., Lindgren, F.T., & Wood, P.D. (1988). Co-ordinate changes in levels of human serum low and high density lipoprotein subclasses in healthy men. *Arteriosclerosis,* **8,** 155–162.

Lapidus, L., Bengtsson, C., Larsson, B., Pennert, K., Rybo, E., & Sjostrom, L. (1984). Distribution of adipose tissue and risk of cardiovascular disease and death: A 12 year follow up of participants in the population study of women in Gothenburg, Sweden. *British Medical Journal,* **289,** 1257–1261.

Lipid Research Clinics Program. (1984). The Lipid Research Clinics Coronary Primary Prevention Trial Results. II. The relationship of reduction in incidence of coronary heart disease to cholesterol lowering. *Journal of the American Medical Association,* **251,** 365–374.

Morris, J.N., Everitt, M.G., Pollard, R., & Chave, S.P.W. (1980). Vigorous exercise in leisure-time: Protection against coronary heart disease. *Lancet,* **2,** 1207–1210.

National Cholesterol Education Program. (1987). Highlights of the report of the expert panel on detection, evaluation, and treatment of high blood cholesterol in adults. NIH Publication No. 88-2926. Bethesda, MD: National Institutes of Health.

Paffenbarger, R.S., Hyde, R.T., Wing, W.L., & Steinmetz, C.H. (1984). A natural history of athleticism and cardiovascular health. *Journal of the American Medical Association,* **252,** 491–495.

Sopko, G., Leon, A.S., Jacobs, D.R., Foster, N., Moy, J., Kuba, K., Anderson, J.T., Casal, D., McNally, C., & Frantz, I. (1985). The effects of exercise and weight loss on plasma lipids in young obese men. *Metabolism,* **34,** 227–236.

Stefanick, M.L., Terry, R.B., Haskell, W.L., & Wood, P.D. (1988). Relationships of changes in post-heparin hepatic and lipoprotein lipase activity to HDL-cholesterol changes following weight loss achieved by dieting versus exercise. In L.L. Gallo (Ed.), *Cardiovascular disease: Molecular and cellular mechanisms. Prevention and treatment* (pp. 61–69). New York: Plenum Press.

Terry, R.B., Stefanick, M.L., Krauss, R.M., Haskell, W.L., & Wood, P.D. (1985). Relationships between abdomen to hip ratio, plasma lipoproteins and sex hormones. *Circulation, 72,* III–452.

Williams, P.T., Krauss, R.M., Wood, P.D., Lindgren, F.T., Giotas, C., & Vranizan, K.M. (1986). Lipoprotein subfractions of runners and sedentary men. *Metabolism, 35,* 45–52.

Wood, P.D., Haskell, W.L., & Fortmann, S.P. (1986). Effects on lipoproteins of weight loss by dieting versus exercise in a controlled trial. *CVD Epidemiology Newsletter, 39,* 50.

Wood, P.D., Terry, R.B., & Haskell, W.L. (1985). Metabolism of substrates: Diet, lipoprotein metabolism, and exercise. *Federation Proceedings, 44,* 358–363.

Wood, P.D., Williams, P.T., & Haskell, W.L. (1984). Physical activity and high-density lipoproteins. In N.E. Miller & G.J. Miller (Eds.), *Clinical and metabolic aspects of high-density lipoproteins* (pp. 135–165). Amsterdam: Elsevier Science.

Effects of Exercise on Biological Features of Aging

Roy J. Shephard

University of Toronto, Ontario, Canada

Biological features of aging may be studied at several levels of organization. We shall here discuss aging of the whole organism, the concepts of overall biological and appraised age, and—as examples of organ and cellular change—the age-related deterioration of function in the oxygen transport system. At all levels of organization, these processes seem susceptible to modification by both disease and habitual exercise (Shephard, 1987).

Aging of the Whole Organism

Animal Experiments

In the whole organism, aging leads to an increased probability of death, as summarized in various types of Gompertz plot. There are several difficulties in testing the influence of habitual activity upon this relationship by a controlled experiment where some animals are exercised regularly and others are assigned a sedentary existence. First, it is difficult to equate either exercise programs or life spans between animals and humans. Does 30 min of running per day provide the same stimulus to a greyhound as a human? Can we compare the responses of a 400-day rat with those of a 40-year-old human? Does a human who takes a 5-km country walk face the same stress as a rat forced to swim in a cold bath by weights tied to its tail or encouraged to run on a treadmill by repeated electrical shocks? It is also difficult to match active and inactive animals in terms of body mass. Edington, Cosmas, and McCafferty (1972) suggested that the life span of rats was extended by daily treadmill running, but only if their exercise program was begun before the age of 400 days; they speculated that by this stage, irreversible effects of a previous sedentary lifestyle had become established. More recently, Holloszy and Smith

(1987) reported that while exercised animals lived longer than sedentary littermates who were allowed to become obese, if animals were matched in terms of body mass, then sedentary animals lived longer than those who were exercised.

Human Experiments

In humans, the shape of the survival curve has become progressively more rectangular in recent years (Fries, 1980). In essence, use of the probability of death as an index of biological aging has been confounded by secular changes in habitual activity and the prevalence of disease. As major sources of illness have been controlled, fewer people have been dying prematurely, but the fundamental aging process has apparently remained unchanged. Excitement over supposedly long-lived and active populations has been exposed as an artifact of age exaggeration among primitive societies (Mazess & Forman, 1979). Comparisons of longevity between former athletes and their nonathletic peers have also proven unsatisfactory, partly because of failure to control for differences of lifestyle between the two types of population and partly because of failure to ascertain current activity patterns among those classified as athletes (Montoye, Van Huss, Olson, Pierson, & Hudec, 1957; Polednak, 1978; Shephard, 1987; Yamaji & Shephard, 1978).

However, the Harvard alumni study (Paffenbarger, Hyde, Wing, & Hsieh, 1986) has found up to a 2-year increase of life span in those men who continue to expend 8 megajoules (MJ) per week in deliberate leisure activity, and this advantage over their sedentary peers persists after correction for other risk factors such as blood pressure status, cigarette smoking, net gain in body mass since college, and age of parental death. Presumably, those in the active group have won these gains by a squaring of their personal aging curve, as the likelihood of premature death from cardiovascular disease has been reduced, although there is as yet no evidence that their intrinsic patterns of aging have been changed.

Shephard and Montelpare (1988) recently carried out a retrospective survey on a substantial sample of people 65 years of age and older. Subjects were asked to report their habitual activity at the age of 50 years, on the basis that adult leisure patterns had stabilized by this age. Study participants were then divided into three categories on the basis of their reported activity (Table 1); among the men, there was no evidence that a greater proportion of those who reported a high level of activity survived to the highest age categories, but in women a greater proportion of those reporting moderate activity appeared to survive to the highest ages ($p <$ 0.05). Moreover, in the active subjects of both sexes, there was a significant trend to less restriction of activity and thus a better quality of life in the retirement years (Table 2).

Biological Age, Appraised Age and the Aging of Organ Function

Biological Age. Because the rate of aging varies from one organ to another, gerontologists have attempted to develop formulas that pool a variety of anthropometric, physiologic, and psychologic measures to yield

Table 1   The Influence of Habitual Activity at the Age of 50 Years on Subsequent Survival

Current age quintile	Proportion of subjects		
	Active (score 2.0–38.0 units)	Moderately active (score 2.0–20.9 units)	Vigorously active (score 21.0–38.0 units)
65–69	0.84	0.61	0.23
70–74	0.85	0.61	0.23
74–79	0.76	0.52	0.26
80–84	0.80	0.59	0.23
85+	0.82	0.59	0.23

Note. Subjects classified according to arbitrary activity scale; significant age gradient ($p < .05$) for women reporting moderate activity. Data from "Geriatric Benefits of Exercise as an Adult" by R.J. Shephard and W. Montelpare, 1988, *Journal of Gerontology,* **43**, pp. M86–M90.

Table 2   The Influence of Habitual Activity at the Age of 50 Years on the Quality of Life During the Retirement Years

Current disability	Mean activity at age 50 yr (arbitrary units)	*SD*	*n*
None	9.28	9.76	286
Minor	8.12	8.94	126
Severe limitation	7.70	9.43	173
Institutionalized	4.06	6.63	25

Note. See data note to Table 1.

a biologic age for a given individual (Bourlière, 1982; Comfort, 1969; Heikkinen, 1979). However, if the proposed data, such as standing height, hair graying, maximum voluntary ventilation, visual acuity, and autoantibody titers are subjected to a factor analysis, there is no evidence that a single "general aging" component emerges. Indeed, it is difficult to envisage why such a diverse range of biological processes should deteriorate at a common rate in any given person, and the loss of function in individual organs is often better correlated with calendar age than with a biological age derived from a pooling of the available data on aging.

Appraised Age.   Given that one possible definition of aging is an increased probability of death, the gerontologist may find more use for the concept of "appraised age" than for that of "biological age." The Canadian version of the Health Hazard Appraisal procedure was developed by Health and Welfare Canada (1976) and Spasoff, McDowell, Wright, and Dunkeley (1980). Risk-taking behavior is reported on a simple questionnaire, and a "composite risk score" is computed for each subject. This takes account of the chances of dying from each of the 12 principal causes of death over the next 10 years. An "appraised age" is then presented, which is the age of a population having the same probability of dying as the individual under consideration. Calculations are repeated with all modifiable risk factors reduced to the recommended level; this yields an "achievable risk" for the individual and a corresponding "achievable" or "compliance" age.

We applied this approach to workers volunteering for an employee fitness program (Shephard, Corey, & Cox, 1983). As anticipated, the group was already somewhat health conscious, with an initial appraised age that was lower than their calendar age (an advantage of 3.1 years in female subjects and 1.8 years in male subjects). Nevertheless, there was still some scope for a reduction of risk-taking behavior, particularly in the men, the gap between the appraised and the compliance age amounting to 1.7 years in females and 3.8 years in males. After 6 months' involvement in the fitness program, the gap between the appraised and the compliance age narrowed to 1.4 years in the women and 3.0 years in the men, the development being particularly marked among males with high adherence to the program (Table 3).

Organ Function.   Deterioration in many of the individual body systems can become sufficient to limit overall function as years advance, but

Table 3   Relationship Between Compliance With Employee Exercise Program and Change in "appraised age," as Assessed by the Canadian Health Hazard Appraisal

Subject group	Change of appraised age over 6 months (years)	Gain of appraised age (years)
Control subjects	+0.48	+0.02
Experimental subjects		
Nonparticipants	+1.07	−1.57
Dropouts	−0.26	+0.76
Low-adherents	+0.05	+0.45
High-adherents	−0.76	+1.26

Note. Data from "Health Hazard Appraisal—The Influence of an Employee Fitness Programme" by R.J. Shephard, P. Corey, and M. Cox, 1982, *Canadian Journal of Public Health,* **73**, 183–187.

recently particular interest has focused on the progressive decrease in oxygen transport. Unfortunately, several pieces of evidence show that aging of the oxygen transport system is closely intertwined with changes attributable to disease and alterations in habitual activity. Some years ago, Brown and Shephard (1967) noted that about a quarter of older female employees of a department store were affected by some form of chronic disease that impaired oxygen transport, and the maximum oxygen intake of this subsample was 10% to 14% below that of other workers. Again, in a large cross-sectional survey of the Saskatoon population, information was collected on habitual activity patterns. It was noted that the line describing the aging of oxygen transport in the active members of the community ran parallel with that for those who were sedentary, although the former was set at a higher level (Bailey, Shephard, Mirwald, & McBride, 1974). Finally, a 10-year longitudinal study of an Inuit community in the course of acculturation to a North American lifestyle showed a substantial deterioration of maximum oxygen intake at all ages as the population became physically less active (Rode & Shephard, 1984; Figure 1).

Until recently, the explanation of the age-related decline in oxygen transport seemed relatively simple: There was a progressive decline in the main determinant of maximum oxygen transport, the maximum cardiac output (Niinimaa & Shephard, 1978). However, it is now argued that the decline in maximum oxygen intake, for all its regularity of slope in many different populations, is partly an artifact of declining habitual activity (Heath, Hagberg, Ehsani, & Holloszy, 1981). Moreover, some authors such as Lakatta, Mitchell, Pomerance, and Rowe (1987) have experienced difficulty in defining a traditional oxygen consumption plateau when testing elderly patients, and they have argued from this that the peak of aerobic function is limited by difficulty in shunting cardiac output to the exercising limbs, an inadequate muscle mass, or some other noncardiac factor. Rodeheffer et al. (1984) have further postulated that if subjects with ischemic changes in the myocardium are excluded by a combination of exercise electrocardiography and scintigraphy, the classical age-related decrease of maximum cardiac output is not observed; rather, the Frank-Starling mechanism is invoked, so that an increased end-diastolic volume and maximum stroke volume compensate for the lower maximal heart rate of the older subjects.

Can additional inferences about the deterioration of oxygen transport with age be drawn from performance data? The performance in many endurance events, including cross-country skiing, distance swimming, and distance running, deteriorates regularly over the span of adult life (Rahe & Arthur, 1975; Riegel, 1981; Stones & Kozma, 1980). Because there is little change in the mechanical efficiency of running as a person becomes older, it is tempting to deduce that there has been a corresponding loss of oxygen transport (about 1% per year in men). The weakness in this argument is that a constant level of competition is assumed at all ages, when in fact competition is much more keen among those in the younger age groups. This problem is highlighted by extending the analysis

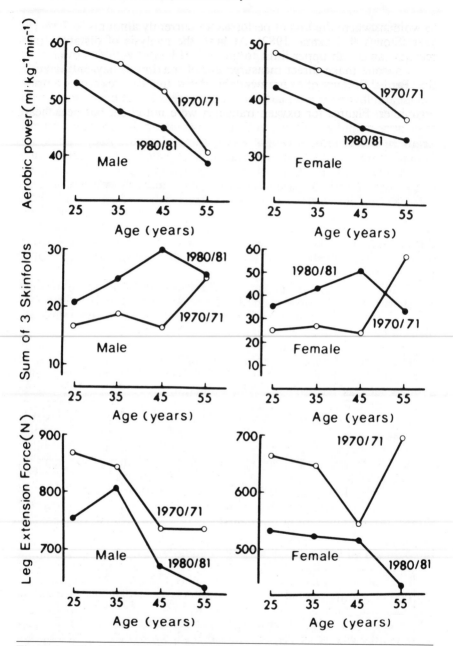

Figure 1.   The influence of acculturation to an urban North American lifestyle upon the aging of maximum oxygen intake, body fat, and muscle strength. Data from "Ten Years of 'Civilization'—Fitness of Canadian Inuit" by A. Rode and R.J. Shephard, 1984, *Journal of Applied Physiology, Respiratory, Environmental and Exercise Physiology,* **56,** 1472–1477.

to women, where the loss of performance currently amounts to 2.5% per year (Stones & Kozma, 1982). At best, the analysis of distance track records can set an upper limit to the rate of loss of aerobic power.

Can one make direct measurement of maximum oxygen intake in the elderly? Because of a commendable desire to measure cardiac output, Lakatta et al. (1987) studied "maximum voluntary exercise" on a cycle ergometer. Figures for oxygen transport were not cited, but peak heart rates were quite low relative to the anticipated maximum values for the age groups under investigation. Even young adults may experience difficulties in reaching a well-defined plateau of oxygen consumption on a cycle ergometer. During this type of exercise, a large part of the muscular effort is sustained by a quadriceps muscle, which contracts at a high percentage of its maximum voluntary force; the resultant external vascular impedance presents a prohibitive afterload to the aging heart, and effort is halted by a local accumulation of lactic acid before the maximum cardiac output has been reached (Kay & Shephard, 1969). On the other hand, treadmill testing allows a satisfactory measurement of maximum oxygen intake into the ninth decade of life (Sidney & Shephard, 1977a). Three quarters of elderly subjects reach the classical definition of an oxygen consumption plateau during their first evaluation; in at least half of the remaining individuals, a plateau is reached with a second attempt, and in the remaining subjects ancillary evidence such as heart rate, respiratory gas exchange ratio, and blood lactate concentrations confirms that a true maximum effort has been realized.

Hollmann (1965) and Dehn and Bruce (1972) argued that the age-related loss of aerobic power was less in continuing athletes than in the general population. However, the figures that they cited for athletes (an annual loss of 0.70 and 0.56 ml $\cdot$ kg^{-1} $\cdot$ min^{-1}, respectively) did not differ substantially from the rate of loss seen in the general North American population, some 9% per decade (Shephard, 1987). Heath et al. (1981) compared 16 Masters athletes with 16 younger competitors, matched on the basis of training distance, training intensity, and best performance at comparable ages; their calculations suggested that active subjects had lost only 5% of aerobic power per decade, an amount that could be attributed simply to the age-related decline in maximum heart rate. Kavanagh and Shephard (1977) found that the average training distance in their sample of Masters competitors was almost identical for the youngest category (average age 34.8 years) and those aged 60 to 70 years; the corresponding decline in aerobic power was only 2.8 ml $\cdot$ kg^{-1} $\cdot$ min^{-1} per decade over a 28.8 year span. Training distances were also comparable between the 40- to 50-year and 50- to 60-year age groups, this part of their sample showing a decrease in peak oxygen intake of 3.8 ml $\cdot$ kg^{-1} $\cdot$ min^{-1} over a 10.3-year span. This order of loss, which has recently been confirmed by the same authors in a much larger sample of Masters athletes, agrees quite closely with the estimate of 3.2 ml $\cdot$ kg^{-1} $\cdot$ min^{-1} hypothesized by Heath et al. and the figure of 3.1 ml $\cdot$ kg^{-1} $\cdot$ min^{-1} per decade observed by Pollock (1974).

In contrast, Saltin (1986) described a loss of 7.3 ml $\cdot$ kg^{-1} $\cdot$ min^{-1} per decade in "still active" orienteers. There are three possible explanations for this apparently conflicting finding: (a) The initial aerobic power of Saltin's group was much higher (81 ml · kg^{-1} · min^{-1} as young adults), (b) the initial age of the orienteers was greater (the span was from 55 to 75 years), and (c) a possible age-related decrease in the weekly training distance was not excluded. We may conclude that in most cross-sectional studies of athletes where the habitual activity of the subjects has remained constant from one age category to another, the loss of aerobic power has been somewhat less than in the general population (where the true rate of aging is exaggerated by an associated decline of habitual activity); nevertheless, the maximum oxygen intake of the athletes does diminish by 2.8 to 3.8 ml · kg^{-1} · min^{-1} per decade (5–6%).

Determinants of Maximum Oxygen Intake

In some older people, effort is halted short of a traditional oxygen consumption plateau because of breathlessness. However, the reasons usually reported for halting a maximum test (weak muscles, poor coordination, or impending loss of consciousness) reflect an inadequate cardiac output rather than respiratory failure.

Various manifestations of myocardial ischemia (anginal pain, premature ventricular contractions, and deep ST segmental depression) limit oxygen transport in a proportion of subjects over the age of 40 (Montoye, 1975; Sidney & Shephard, 1977b). Participation in a program of regular endurance exercise should reduce myocardial oxygen demand at any given power output (because the pulse-pressure product is lower), and it may also improve coronary perfusion (because the diastolic phase of the cardiac cycle becomes relatively longer). However, both of these theoretical advantages of training tend to be lost during a maximal effort test, and in practice the proportion of Masters athletes with abnormal electrocardiographic (ECG) records during all-out exercise is similar to that in sedentary subjects (Gibbons, Cooper, Martin, & Pollock, 1977; Grimby & Saltin, 1966; Kavanagh & Shephard, 1977). In a recent large survey of older competitors, we found 10.9% exercise ECG abnormalities in those aged 30 to 39, and in subsequent decades there were 13.8%, 20.4%, 27.5% and 29.6% abnormal records. Some of these are "false positive" responses, but at least it is clear that myocardial ischemia is a factor in no more than 20% to 25% of older competitors; in the remaining 75% to 80%, oxygen intake is limited by cardiac pump function rather than exercise-induced ischemia.

Cardiac Function

Maximal cardiac output is determined by the product of heart rate, arteriovenous oxygen difference, and stroke volume. In the sedentary adult, the maximum heart rate declines from about 195 beats · min^{-1} at the age of 25 years to around 170 beats · min^{-1} at the age of 65 (Sidney & Shephard, 1977a), a loss of some 6.3% per decade. Training gives some decrease of maximum heart rate at any age, but nevertheless the age-related decrease of heart rate in an active individual is similar to that observed in a sedentary person (Saltin, 1986).

The arteriovenous oxygen difference of older adults is normal or even increased in submaximal effort, but the maximum arteriovenous oxygen difference is reduced by about 10% relative to that anticipated in younger individuals (Niinimaa & Shephard, 1978; Shephard, 1987). The elderly are not generally anemic, and the arterial oxygen content is well maintained; nor are there changes in muscle capillarity or tissue enzyme activity that restrict oxygen extraction. Saltin (1986) found a femoral venous oxygen content of only 18 ml $\cdot$ L^{-1} in elderly orienteers, compared with 25 ml $\cdot$ L^{-1} in their younger peers. By elimination of other possibilities, the narrowed arteriovenous oxygen difference of the older person thus reflects a partial failure of the body to redirect blood flow from the inactive muscles, viscera, and skin to the working tissues (Shephard, 1987).

The well-trained athlete loses less muscle mass than a sedentary person with aging. Because of less thickness of subcutaneous fat and more ready sweating, the active individual also has less need to direct blood flow to the skin during exercise. However, such differences are more likely to be important during prolonged submaximal effort than in maximum exercise, and both Grimby, Nilsson and Saltin (1966) and Saltin (1986) have observed a relatively low maximum arteriovenous oxygen difference (134 ml $\cdot$ L^{-1}) in older orienteers.

In 1981, Heath et al. claimed that the oxygen pulse (the product of arteriovenous oxygen difference and stroke volume) did not decline with age. If supported, this observation would suggest that the age-related reduction of arteriovenous oxygen difference had been compensated by an increase of stroke volume. Two weaknesses in their cross-sectional study of runners were pointed out by Saltin (1986); to judge from maximum oxygen intakes, the young comparison group were not elite performers, and because exercise blood pressures were no higher in the older than in the younger group, it is debatable whether the former reached maximum effort (where stroke volume might have been impaired by an increase of afterload). Hagberg et al. (1985) later revised their opinion on oxygen pulse; the 1985 report indicated a small decline with age. Saltin (1986) also found a decline of oxygen pulse from 0.42 ml $\cdot$ kg^{-1} $\cdot$ beat^{-1} at 26 years to 0.32 ml $\cdot$ kg^{-1} $\cdot$ beat^{-1} at the age of 66 years, the 23.8% change reflecting both a decrease of arteriovenous oxygen difference and a decrease of maximum stroke volume. Even in the "six best" orienteers, who were said to be increasing their training schedule, there was still an age-related decrease of both maximum oxygen intake and oxygen pulse; the final figure for the six was 0.32 ml $\cdot$ kg^{-1} $\cdot$ beat^{-1}, a value comparable with the average for the group.

Rodeheffer et al. (1984) and Lakatta et al. (1987) have argued that much of the supposed deterioration of cardiac function with age is due to subclinical disease. Certainly, the onset of severe myocardial ischemia can cause a decline of stroke volume and even cardiac failure (Parker, diGiorgi, & West, 1966), but it is less clear that the moderate, exercise-induced ECG changes seen in 25% of older athletes have a similar effect. Moreover, the concept of restricting analyses to an elderly population where no one shows minor electrocardiographic or scintigraphic changes is somewhat artificial. The data also show considerable scatter, and for technical reasons the Baltimore investigators were unable to take their subjects to the usually accepted criteria of maximum performance (where they, like other investigators, might have observed a restriction of stroke volume).

Maximum cardiac outputs for the younger subjects of the Baltimore series appear relatively low, whereas if the reported stroke volumes of the elderly are multiplied by generally accepted maximum heart rates for the elderly, the resultant cardiac outputs imply that the older age categories had either an unrealistically large maximum oxygen intake or an unrealistically low arteriovenous oxygen difference. Unfortunately, Lakatta et al. (1987) have provided no information on either of these last two variables. Finally, their own data show that although the adverse effect of age upon the exercise-related increase of cardiac ejection fraction (Port, Cobb, Coleman, & Jones, 1980; Schocken, Blumenthal, Port, Hindle, & Coleman, 1983) is less after exclusion of patients with myocardial ischemia, nevertheless many subjects in the age range 60 to 80 years demonstrate little or no increase over their resting ejection fraction during vigorous effort (Rodeheffer et al., 1984).

Grimby et al. (1966) found that in 51-year-old orienteers, the maximum cardiac output was 5 L $\cdot$ min^{-1}, 17% lower than in their 25-year-old peers. Although much of this difference was due to a decrease of maximal heart rate, there was also a small decrease of maximal stroke volume. As noted above, more recent data on the oxygen pulse of older competitors (Saltin, 1986) support this view.

The mean systemic blood pressure rises progressively with age both at rest and during exercise (Hanson, Tabakin, Levy, & Nedde, 1968). Moreover, although regular training can induce a therapeutically useful decrease of resting blood pressure (Tipton, 1984), during maximum effort well-trained subjects develop a larger cardiac output and thus as high a final blood pressure as their sedentary counterparts (Saltin, 1986). If stroke volume is well maintained in the face of this increased pressure, there must be adaptive changes in the myocardium. Linzbach and Akuamoa-Boateng (1973) suggested that between the ages of 30 and 90 years, heart mass increased by 1 g $\cdot$ yr^{-1} in men and 1.5 g $\cdot$ yr^{-1} in women. Likewise, Kavanagh and Shephard (1977) found that the radiographic heart volume of Masters athletes was sustained and even increased among older members of their sample. Echocardiographic data confirm a moderate age-related increase of left ventricular wall thickness in both systole and diastole (Gerstenblith et al., 1977; Nishimura, Yamada, & Kawai, 1980; Sjogren, 1971). The increase of mass seems due largely to an increase in average myocyte size (Unverferth, Fetters, & Unverferth, 1983), although there is also some accumulation of both collagen and amyloid (Hodkinson & Pomerance, 1977).

However, it has yet to be established that the age-related increase of cardiac mass is effective in increasing stroke volume. Function could be adversely influenced by a decrease of preloading, an increase of after-loading, or a decrease of ventricular power. Structural deteriorations in the venous system, together with a decrease of total blood volume and poor tone in the capacity vessels, reduce preloading in an older person, and these problems are exacerbated by a decrease of ventricular compliance, with delayed relaxation of the heart wall, at least in early diastole (Gerstenblith et al., 1977; Lakatta et al., 1987). Afterloading is increased by the greater volume of blood to be accelerated in a distended aorta and less distensibility of the sclerosed arterial walls (O'Rourke, 1982). At the same time, atrophied muscles are forced to contract at a higher fraction of their maximum voluntary force to sustain a given power output, and systemic blood pressure rises in an attempt to sustain perfusion of the active limbs (Kay & Shephard, 1969).

Finally, much of the required increase of stroke volume during exercise is mediated by an increase of myocardial contractility. With aging, there is a decrease of beta-receptor sensitivity or density that reduces the inotropic response of the myocytes to a standard dose of catecholamine (Lakatta, 1980), although an older person tends to compensate for this potential handicap by a greater increase of catecholamine levels during vigorous exercise (Ziegler, Lake, & Kopin, 1976). The aging heart muscle certainly takes longer to develop peak force; however, a slowing of Ca^{2+} sequestration by the sarcoplasmic reticulum is involved (Froelich, Lakatta, & Beard, 1978), in addition to any lessening of the normal inotropic response to catecholamines.

Research Challenges

The examples provided here illustrate a continuing challenge to gerontology: distinguishing the inherent rate of aging from the impact of age-related environmental influences, including the effects of disease, changing patterns of habitual activity, and other aspects of personal lifestyle. There is a necessary division between pure gerontology and its applied counterpart that considers the responses of an older person living in a real world where the environment is almost inevitably less than ideal. The discrepancy between these two impressions of the aging process poses a challenge to preventive medicine. How far can our current environment be modified to approximate the actual course of aging to its "pure" potential? In the specific context of regular physical activity, the studies of Paffenbarger et al. (1986) need to be confirmed and extended, exploring why the mortality of an older human apparently reacts more favorably than that of an experimental animal if the level of habitual activity is increased (Tables 4 and 5).

There is a need to define more closely an optimum pattern of activity that will extend the period of human survival. Responses to enhanced exercise should be compared at various levels of other current risk factors,

Table 4   Added Life from an Active Lifestyle (Leisure Energy Expenditure >8 MJ/wk vs. <2 MJ/wk)

Age (yr)	Gain of life expectancy (yr)	
	Crude	Adjusted[a]
35–39	2.64	2.51
55–59	2.25	2.02
65–69	1.64	1.35
75–79	0.35	0.42

Note. Data from "Physical Activity, All Cause Mortality and Longevity of College Alumni" by R.S. Paffenbarger, R.T. Hyde, A.L. Wing, and C.C. Hsieh, 1986, *New England Journal of Medicine,* **314**, 605–613.

[a]Adjusted for differences in blood pressure status, cigarette smoking, net gain in body mass index since college, and age of parental death, as reported on entry to the study.

Table 5   Influence of Type of Physical Activity on Relative Risk of Death

Level of activity	Walking	Stair climbing	Playing light sports	Playing vigorous sports
Low	1.00	1.00	1.00	1.00
Moderate	0.85	0.85	0.76	0.65
High	0.79	0.92	0.70	0.74

Note. The optimum weekly prescription is walking >15 km, climbing 350–1049 stairs, playing >3 hr of light sports or 1 to 2 hr of vigorous sports. (See data note to Table 4.)

and observations should be continued beyond "young" old age into the period of "inevitable" death (80–100 years). However, we must also remember that the quality of life is of greater importance to most senior citizens than its duration. Thus work is urgently needed on the relative importance of the various factors that restrict function during the years of retirement and on the extent to which these limitations can be avoided by a change of personal lifestyle.

Substantial differences of chronology, pathology, and lifestyle between animals and humans will necessitate a continued focus of exercise and aging research upon human rather than animal models. Investigators may occasionally gain the support needed for long-term experimental studies, but it seems likely that the resultant data will lack general applicability because of subject selection—both initially and through poor compliance with assigned regimens. The main source of new information will thus be painstaking and costly epidemiological observations. The emphasis of such studies will shift increasingly from mere calculations of survival rates to assessments of life quality and the demand for institutional or medical support; in this fashion, an answer will be provided for those who argue that an extension of life span will increase rather than decrease geriatric costs.

Acknowledgment

The gerontological studies of this laboratory are supported in part by a research development grant from the University of Toronto.

References

Bailey, D.A., Shephard, R.J., Mirwald, R.L., & McBride, G.A. (1974). A current view of cardiorespiratory fitness levels of Canadians. *Canadian Medical Association Journal, III,* 25–30.

Bourlière, F. (1982). *Gérontologie: Biologie et clinique.* Paris: Flammarion.

Brown, J.R., & Shephard, R.J. (1967). Some measurements of fitness in older female employees of a Toronto department store. *Canadian Medical Association Journal, 97,* 1208–1213.

Comfort, A. (1969). Test battery to measure ageing rate in man. *Lancet, 2,* 411–414.

Dehn, M., & Bruce, R.A. (1972). Longitudinal variations in maximal oxygen intake with age and activity. *Journal of Applied Physiology, 33,* 805–807.

Edington, D.W., Cosmas, A.C., & McCafferty, W.B. (1972). Exercise and longevity: Evidence for a threshold age. *Journal of Gerontology, 27,* 341–343.

Fries, J.F. (1980). Aging, natural death and the compression of morbidity. *New England Journal of Medicine, 303,* 130–135.

Froelich, J.P., Lakatta, E.G., & Beard, E. (1978). Studies of sarco-plasmic reticulum function and contraction duration in young adult and aged rat myocardium. *Journal of Molecular and Cellular Cardiology, 10,* 427–438.

Gerstenblith, G., Fredericksen, J., Yin, F.C., Fortuin, N.J., Lakatta, E.G., & Weisfeldt, M.L. (1977). Echocardiographic assessment of a normal adult aging population. *Circulation, 56,* 273–278.

Gibbons, L.K., Cooper, K.H., Martin, R.P., & Pollock, M.L. (1977). Medical examination and electrocardiographic analysis of elite distance runners. *Annals of the New York Academy of Sciences, 301,* 283–296.

Grimby, G., & Saltin, B. (1966). Physiological analysis of physically well-trained middle-aged and old athletes. *Acta Medica Scandinavica, 179,* 513–526.

Grimby, G., & Saltin, B. (1971). Physiological effects of physical conditioning. *Scandinavian Journal of Rehabilitation Medicine, 3,* 6–14.

Grimby, G., Nilsson, N.J., & Saltin, B. (1966). Cardiac output during submaximal and maximal exercise in active middle-aged athletes. *Journal of Applied Physiology,* **21,** 1150–1156.

Hagberg, J.M., Allen, W.K., Seals, D.R., Hurley, B.F., Ehsani, A.A., & Holloszy, J.O. (1985). A hemodynamic comparison of young and older endurance athletes during exercise. *Journal of Applied Physiology,* **58,** 2041–2046.

Hanson, J., Tabakin, B., Levy, A., & Nedde, W. (1968). Long-term physical training and cardiovascular dynamics in middle-aged men. *Circulation,* **38,** 783–789.

Health and Welfare, Canada. (1976). Your lifestyle profile—operation lifestyle. Ottawa, ON: Promotion and Prevention Directorate, Health and Welfare, Canada.

Heath, G.W., Hagberg, J.M., Ehsani, A.A., & Holloszy, J.O. (1981). A physiological comparison of young and older endurance athletes. *Journal of Applied Physiology,* **51,** 634–640.

Heikkinen, E. (1979). Normal aging. Definition, problems and relation to physical activity. In H. Orimo, K. Shimada, M. Iriki, and D. Maeda (Eds.), *Recent advances in gerontology* (pp. 501–503). Amsterdam: Excerpta Medica.

Hodkinson, H.M., & Pomerance, A. (1977). The clinical significance of senile cardiac amyloidosis: A prospective clinico-pathological study. *Quarterly Journal of Medicine,* **46,** 381–387.

Hollmann, W. (1965). *Korperliches Training als Pravention von Herz-Kreislauf Krankheiten.* Stuttgart, W. Germany: Hippokrates Verlag.

Holloszy, J.O., & Smith, E.K. (1987). Effects of exercise on longevity of rats. *Federation Proceedings,* **46,** 1850–1853.

Kavanagh, T., & Shephard, R.J. (1977). The effects of continued training on the aging process. *Annals of the New York Academy of Sciences,* **301,** 656–670.

Kay, C., & Shephard, R.J. (1969). On muscle strength and the threshold of anaerobic work. *Internationale Zeitschrift für Angewandte und Arbeitsphysiologie,* **27,** 311–328.

Lakatta, E.G. (1980). Age-related alterations in cardiovascular response to adrenergic mediated stress. *Federation Proceedings,* **39,** 3173–3177.

Lakatta, E.G., Mitchell, J.H., Pomerance, A., & Rowe, G.G. (1987). Human aging: Changes in structure and function. *Journal of the American College of Cardiology,* **10,** 42A–47A.

Linzbach, A.J., & Akuamoa-Boateng, E. (1973). Changes in the aging human heart. I. Heart weight in the aged. *Klinische Wochenschrift,* **51,** 56–163.

Mazess, R.B., & Forman, S.H. (1979). Longevity and age exaggeration in Vilcabamba, Ecuador. *Journal of Gerontology,* **34,** 94–98.

Montoye, H.J. (1975). *Physical activity and health: An epidemiological study of an entire community.* Englewood Cliffs, NJ: Prentice Hall.

Montoye, H.J., Van Huss, W.D., Olson, H., Pierson, W.R., & Hudec, A. (1957). *The longevity and morbidity of college athletes.* Michigan State University: Phi Epsilon Kappa Fraternity.

Niinimaa, V., & Shephard, R.J. (1978). Training and exercise conductance in the elderly: 2. The cardiovascular system. *Journal of Gerontology,* **33,** 362–367.

Nishimura, T., Yamada, Y., & Kawai, C. (1980). Echocardiographic evaluation of long-term effects of exercise on left ventricular hypertrophy and function in professional bicyclists. *Circulation,* **61,** 832–840.

O'Rourke, M.F. (1982). *Aging and arterial function* (pp. 185–195). New York: Churchill Livingstone.

Paffenbarger, R.S., Hyde, R.T., Wing, A.L., & Hsieh, C.C. (1986). Physical activity, all cause mortality and longevity of college alumni. *New England Journal of Medicine,* **314,** 605–613.

Parker, J.O., diGiorgi, S., & West, R.O. (1966). A hemodynamic study of coronary insufficiency precipitated by exercise. With observations on the effects of nitroglycerine. *American Journal of Medicine,* **17,** 470–483.

Polednak, A.P. (1978). *The longevity of athletes.* Springfield, IL: Charles C Thomas.

Pollock, M.L. (1974). Physiological characteristics of older champion track athletes. *Research Quarterly,* **45,** 363–373.

Port, S., Cobb, F.R., Coleman, E., & Jones, R.H. (1980). Effect of age on the response of the left ventricular ejection fraction to exercise. *New England Journal of Medicine,* **303,** 1133–1137.

Rahe, R.H., & Arthur, R.J. (1975). Swim performance decrement over middle life. *Medicine and Science in Sports,* **7,** 53–58.

Riegel, P.S. (1981). Athletic records and human endurance. *American Scientist,* **69,** 285–290.

Rode, A., & Shephard, R.J. (1984). Ten years of "civilization"—fitness of Canadian Inuit. *Journal of Applied Physiology, Respiratory, Environmental and Exercise Physiology,* **56,** 1472–1477.

Rodeheffer, R.J., Gerstenblith, G., Becker, C.C., Fleg, J.L., Weisfeldt, M.L., & Lakatta, E.G. (1984). Exercise cardiac output is maintained with advancing age in healthy human subjects: Cardiac dilatation and increased stroke volume compensation for a diminished heart rate. *Circulation,* **69,** 203–213.

Saltin, B. (1986). Physiological characteristics of the masters athlete. In J.R. Sutton & R.M. Brock (Eds.), *Sports medicine for the mature athlete* (pp. 59–80). Indianapolis: Benchmark Press.

Schocken, D.D., Blumenthal, J.A., Port, S., Hindle, P., & Coleman, R.E. (1983). Physical conditioning and left ventricular performance in the elderly: Assessment by radionuclide angiocardiography. *American Journal of Cardiology,* **52,** 359–364.

Shephard, R.J. (1987). *Physical activity and aging* (2nd ed.). London: Croom Helm.

Shephard, R.J., Corey, P., & Cox, M. (1982). Health hazard appraisal—the influence of an employee fitness programme. *Canadian Journal of Public Health,* **73,** 183–187.

Shephard, R.J., & Montelpare, W. (1988). Geriatric benefits of exercise as an adult. *Journal of Gerontology,* **43,** M86–M90.

Sidney, K.H., & Shephard, R.J. (1977a). Maximum and submaximum exercise tests in men and women in the seventh, eighth and ninth decades of life. *Journal of Applied Physiology,* **43,** 280–287.

Sidney, K.H., & Shephard, R.J. (1977b). Training and e.c.g. abnormalities in the elderly. *British Heart Journal,* **39,** 1114–1120.

Sjogren, A.L. (1971). Left ventricular wall thickness in 100 subjects without heart disease. *Chest,* **60,** 341–346.

Spasoff, R.A., McDowell, I., Wright, P.A., & Dunkeley, G. (1980). Reviewing health hazard appraisal. *Chronic Diseases in Canada,* **1,** 16–17.

Spurgeon, H.A., Steinbach, M.F., & Lakatta, E.G. (1983). Chronic exercise prevents characteristic age-related changes in rat cardiac contraction. *American Journal of Physiology,* **244,** (*Heart and Circulatory Physiology,* **13**), H513–H518.

Stones, M.J., & Kozma, A. (1980). Adult age trends in athletic performances. *Experimental Aging Research,* **7,** 269–280.

Stones, M.J., & Kozma, A. (1982). Sex differences in changes with age in record running performances. *Canadian Journal on Aging,* **1,** 12–16.

Tipton, C.M. (1984). Exercise, training and hypertension. *Exercise and Sports Science Reviews,* **12,** 245–306.

Unverferth, D.V., Fetters, J.K., & Unverferth, B.J. (1983). Human myocardial histologic characteristics in congestive heart failure. *Circulation,* **68,** 1194–1200.

Yamaji, K., & Shephard, R.J. (1978). Longevity and cause of death in athletes: A review of the literature. *Journal of Human Ergology,* **6,** 15–27.

Ziegler, M.G., Lake, C.R., & Kopin, I.J. (1976). Plasma noradrenaline increases with age. *Nature,* **261,** 333–335.

Effects of Exercise on the Immune System: Relationship to Stress

Jay M. Weiss
Duke University Medical Center
Durham, North Carolina

Exercise and Stress

This article is written from the perspective of one who is neither an immunologist nor an authority on effects of physical exercise, but rather one who has spent a number of years investigating stress responses. Recently our laboratory has become interested in the effects of stress on the immune system. This article summarizes in a rather general way the effects of muscular exercise on immune responses, with particular attention to how these relate to effects of stress on immunological responses.

This perspective is hardly idiosyncratic given historical antecedents. In surveying the literature on effects of exercise on immune responses, I was struck by the fact that investigators publishing in this area have often viewed exercise as synonymous with stress, using the terms interchangeably. This assumption seemed to me highly problematic. However, after I reviewed the findings, what seemed at the outset to be a rather naive notion seems instead to possess a surprising and intriguing degree of validity.

Describing first effects of stress on immune responses, in the main investigators have found that stressful conditions suppress immunological responses. In both humans and experimental animals, this consequence has been seen in response to many stressful conditions and has been found to affect such diverse measures as lymphocyte cytotoxicity, phagocytosis, lymphocyte proliferation to a mitogen, neutrophil count, interferon production, salivary IgA, ratio of helper/suppressor lymphocytes, and antibody titers to herpes virus (Bartrop, Luckhurst, Lazarus, Kilch, & Penny, 1977; Cohen-Cole et al., 1981; Glaser, Rice, Speicher, Stout, & Kiecolt-Glaser, 1986; Greene, Betts, Ochitill, Iker, & Douglas, 1978; Jemmott et al., 1983; Jensen, 1968; Joasoo & McKenzie, 1976; Kiecolt-Glaser, Garner, Speicher, Penn, & Glaser, 1984; Kiecolt-Glaser et al., 1986; Kimzey, 1975; Monjan & Collector, 1976; Okimura, Ogawa, & Yamauchi, 1986; Palmblad et al., 1976; Pitkin, 1965; Rasmussen, Marsh, & Brillo, 1957; Solomon, 1969; Wister & Hildermann, 1960).

Effects of Strenuous Exercise

If exercise, like stress, produces immunosuppression, and this is expressed in functional effects, one would expect exercise to increase susceptibility to disease and other negative health consequences. Evidence indicates that this can occur. For example, several studies, both experimental and epidemiological, have shown that after infection with poliomyelitis the host is negatively affected by heavy exercise. Over forty years ago, Levinson, Milzer, and Lewin (1945) showed that if during the incubation period of poliomyelitis virus monkeys were forced to swim until exhausted, they developed a higher incidence of and more severe paralysis than did nonexercised subjects. In 1950, Horstman correlated the amount of physical activity and severity of resulting illnesses in 411 patients from three epidemics of poliomyelitis. If around the time of onset of illness physical activity was performed, significant increases in incidence and severity of paralysis were found. Also, a higher percentage of nonparalytic than paralytic patients had a history of bed rest or minimal activity during early stages of the major illness. Similar findings were reported in a clinical survey by Weinstein (1973), who argued that the high incidence of paralysis in males in a community epidemic of polio was related to the fact that all were engaged in strenuous sports.

This observation is not restricted to susceptibility to poliomyelitis. For example, Reyes and Lerner (1976) reported that mice infected with coxsackievirus developed considerably more symptoms and a higher rate of mortality if the animals were strongly exercised during experimental infection with the virus. Beginning on the 14th day of life, half of the mice were swum for 30 min twice a day. Shortly after initiation of the exercise program, all of the mice were infected with coxsackievirus B-3. Viremias and virus in the hearts of exercised mice reached levels that were, respectively, 75 times and 1,000 times greater than in infected but nonexercised mice. At 24 hr after inoculation, serum from the mice that had been swum contained no circulating interferon, whereas infected mice that were not swum had measurable levels of interferon, indicating an immediate immune response to the virus in nonswum animals. At 72 hr after infection, circulating interferon disappeared from animals that were not swum but continued to be present in high titers through the 6th day in mice forced to swim, presumably indicating an ongoing infection in the swum mice.

In summary, literature provides us with several instances in which physical exercise, and particularly large amounts of exercise, is positively correlated with the severity of symptoms following infection with viruses in both man and animals.

Concerning the cellular immunological responses that might constitute the mechanism by which susceptibility to viruses and other pathogenic agents come to express themselves as the diseases described above, a number of studies have examined the effects of physical exercise on immunological responses. As an example, a study by Eskola et al. (1978) assessed the effects of severe exercise on lymphocyte mitogenesis as well as antibody formation to an antigenic challenge. These investigators studied the effects of running a marathon on these measures. Following the marathon, the ability of plasma lymphocytes to respond to three mitogens (PHA, Con A, and PPD) in vitro was found to be significantly decreased (see Figure 1). Antibody formation to a tetanus toxin vaccination given immediately after the marathon, however, was not found to be suppressed 15 days after the vaccination. Thus, a measure of cellular immune responsivity, the ability of T-cells to reproduce to various mitogens, was found to be suppressed by a large amount of physical exercise.

Is Immunosuppression Produced by Elevated Steroids?

An aspect of the paper by Eskola et al. (1978) that is worthy of comment concerns their discussion of potential hormonal mediators for the immunosuppressive effects that they found to result from heavy exercise. These investigators measured considerably elevated levels of circulating steroids in their marathon runners following the race, and much of their discussion concerned the potential role of steroids in mediating the suppression of T-cell mitogenesis that they observed, although they noted

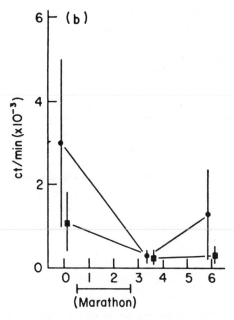

Figure 1.   Effects of marathon running on lymphocyte transformation induced by PPD, 1.0 μg/ml (circles) and 100 μg/ml (squares). The mean and standard error are shown. From "Effect of Sport Stress on Lymphocyte Transformation and Antibody Formation" by J. Eskola, O. Ruuskanen, E. Soppi, M.K. Viljanen, M. Jarvinen, H. Toivonen, and K. Kouvalainen, 1978, *Clinical Experimental Immunology*, **32**, 339–345. Reprinted by permission.

that the evidence was not convincing that steroids mediated this effect. Many investigators have been concerned with the role of circulating steroids in producing immunosuppression, and it was often assumed that these circulating hormones were probably responsible for stress-induced immunosuppression. Consequently, it is worth noting that there is now conclusive evidence, at least in experimental animals whose circulating steroids can be greatly altered, that stress-induced immunosuppression cannot be attributed solely to elevated steroids.

In a series of studies, Keller and colleagues initially showed that exposure of rats to a 19-hr session of uncontrollable electric shocks resulted in profound suppression of T-cell mitogenesis to PHA (Keller, Weiss, Schleifer, Miller, & Stein, 1981). In a subsequent study, these investigators (Keller, Weiss, Schleifer, Miller, & Stein, 1983) then showed that similar effects were obtained in animals that were adrenalectomized prior to stress procedures. This second study included four different groups of hormonally manipulated rats: normal nonoperated, adrenalectomized, sham-operated, and adrenalectomized with a steroid pellet implanted that secreted a constant amount of corticosterone into the circulatory system. The results show that stress-induced suppression of T-cell mitogenesis to PHA occurred in all four groups of animals (Figure 2). As expected, both normal and sham-operated animals showed evidence of decreasing T-cell mitogenesis as the severity of the stressor to which they were exposed increased. In addition, a similar depression of T-cell mitogenesis occurred in both adrenalectomized animals and animals that had a constant low level of circulating corticosterone because of the steroid pellet implant.

Thus, suppression of the ability of T-cells to respond to a mitogen was seen in animals that had no ability to secrete corticosterone (or, in fact, epinephrine either) in response to stressful conditions (i.e., suppression of mitogenesis was seen in both adrenalectomized animals and animals having a fixed circulating level of steroids [via pellet implant]). Interestingly, this study did provide clear evidence that, at least in the rat, the number of circulating lymphocytes (as opposed to responsivity of lymphocytes to a mitogen) was indeed determined by circulating steroid level; both normal and sham-operated animals had markedly decreased numbers of circulating lymphocytes compared with the adrenalectomized animals, whereas the pellet-implanted animals showed a moderate decrease in circulating lymphocytes commensurate with the low level of steroids found in their circulation. The conclusions of this study were (a) that in addition to the effect of adrenal hormones, other hormones or neural mechanisms are quite capable of producing suppression of the T-cell mitogenesis when an animal is exposed to a stressful condition and (b) that it is incorrect to assume that steroids are the principal, or only, mediator of this response when an animal is exposed to stressful conditions. Consequently, preoccupation with stress-induced circulating steroids as the likely mediator for suppression of various cellular immune responses is unwarranted.

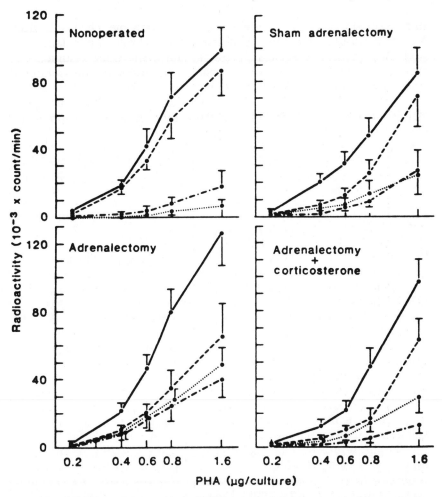

Figure 2.   Effect of stressors in nonoperated, sham-operated, adrenalectomized, and adrenalectomized with pellet implant groups. Stressor conditions are home cage control (solid line), apparatus control (dashed line), low shock (dash and dotted line), and high shock (dotted line). Shown above is mean response (and standard error) of an equivalent number of peripheral blood lymphocytes from each group to PHA stimulation at various doses. From "Stress-Induced Suppression of Immunity in Adrenalectomized Rats" by S.E. Keller, J.M. Weiss, S.J. Schleifer, N.E. Miller, and M. Stein, 1983, *Science,* **221,** 1301–1304. Copyright 1983 by the AAAS.

Effects of Moderate Exercise

The study by Eskola et al. (1978) reported another interesting observation: namely, that although running a marathon suppressed T-cell mitogenesis, exercise of considerably less severity (a 7-km run) had no such suppressant effect—in fact, this exercise slightly elevated the T-cell mitogenic response. Results consistent with this can be seen in other studies of exercise. Targan, Britvan and Dorey (1981) exposed human subjects to very brief exercise (5 min of pedaling on a bicycle ergometer). They reported that this mild exercise regimen elevated the activity of natural killer (NK) cells. Brahmi, Thomas, Park, Park, and Dowdeswell (1985) found similar results, testing individuals again on a cycle ergometer for short periods of time and also testing individuals who had undergone physical exercise conditioning prior to the test. In this study, subjects exercised to 75% of their maximum oxygen consumption, and under these conditions nonconditioned (untrained) male and female subjects exercised on the ergometer for an average of 11.8 minutes, whereas conditioned male subjects exercised for 17.9 minutes. Figure 3 shows that NK cell activity was elevated in both trained and untrained subjects immediately after the exercise. Thus, mild or moderate exercise has the immediate effect of elevating NK cell activity.

Watson et al. (1985) examined another important variable in determining effects of exercise on cellular immune responses—chronicity of the exercise regimen. Thus, these investigators examined the effects of physical conditioning on cellular immune responses. Subjects in this study underwent 15 weeks of exercise training, with training consisting of approximately 1 hr of walking, jogging, and running 5 days per week. After 15 weeks, NK cell activity was found to be somewhat suppressed, but T-cell mitogenesis was markedly elevated relative to a baseline measured 15 weeks prior to the exercise conditioning procedure. It is important to note that the blood sampling in this experiment was not done immediately following one of the exercise sessions, which probably accounts for why NK cell activity was not elevated in this study as it was in the two studies reported in the previous paragraph.

Similar results to those reported by Watson et al. have been seen in experiments using animals as subjects. Fernandes, Rozek, and Troyer (1986) studied the effects of exercising rats for 180 days on a treadmill. The investigators also examined the effect of limiting food intake. The experiment was conducted using spontaneously hypertensive rats (SHR) and their appropriate control subjects (Wistar Kyoto strain). The results showed that T-cell mitogenesis to PHA and Con A was markedly elevated in animals exposed to either the exercise or the diet and was even more elevated in animals exposed to both. Incidentally, a similar effect was found measuring development of hypertension, with exercise and diet preventing the development of hypertension and both manipulations having the most beneficial effect.

Cellular immune responses are regulated to a considerable extent by various soluble factors released by macrophages and lymphocytes. These substances, called interleukins, have also been studied in a preliminary manner in relation to exercise. Cannon and Dinarello (1984) found that human subjects who exercised for approximately 1 hr on a bicycle ergometer evidenced increased levels of interleukin-1 in plasma. Viti, Muscettola, Paulesu, Bocci, and Almi (1985) showed that a similar exercise

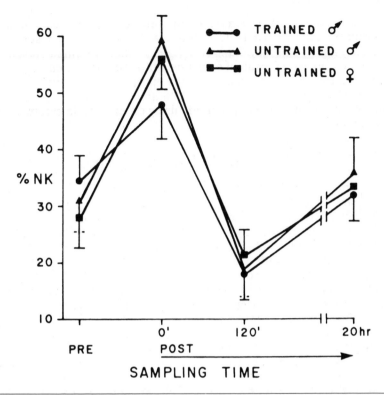

Figure 3.   Average natural killer-cell activity for different groups at four sampling times. The ratio EC:TC was 20:1. The mean and standard error is shown. From "The Effect of Acute Exercise on Natural Killer-Cell Activity of Trained and Sedentary Human Subjects" by Z. Brahmi, J.E. Thomas, M. Park, M. Park, and I.R. Dowdeswell, 1985, *Journal of Clinical Immunology,* **5,** 321–328. Reprinted by permission.

regimen (in which people pedaled until they reached 70% of their aerobic capacity) significantly increased plasma interferon. Thus, acute effects of exercise elevate soluble factors that would, in general, potentiate immune responses. Alteration of these soluble factors is likely to be an important participant in the cellular responses described earlier.

Summary

Looking at this body of data, what general conclusions can one draw? Certain observations seem clear and straightforward. First, severe strenuous exercise markedly depresses a variety of immune parameters and results in increased susceptibility to viral infection and its consequences; this occurs both in individuals who have undergone prolonged exercise conditioning (i.e., marathon runners) and in those who are less well conditioned. Second, exercise that is not too intense or strenuous in nature—for example, exercise for 15 to 60 minutes on a bicycle ergometer or a 30 to 60 minute run or jog—enhances various cellular immune responses, and this occurs in physically conditioned individuals as well as nonconditioned ones. Third, exercise regimens that result in conditioning tend to increase tolerance for exercise such that beneficial effects on immune responses can be obtained with higher amounts of exercise in conditioned individuals.

Relationship of Exercise to Stress

It is of considerable interest that fundamental effects like those just described appear to characterize the relationship between stressful conditions (called "stressors") and immune responses. If one examines the effects of "classical" stressors that have been applied to animals under experimental conditions, one finds effects similar to those previously described occurring with exercise; that is, (a) severe stress results in immunosuppression, (b) moderate stress can result in immunoenhancement, and (c) chronic stress (the equivalent of exercise training resulting in physical conditioning) tends to blunt immunosuppressive effects and can produce immunoenhancement.

The data shown in Figure 4 will serve as a prototypical example of the first two points. These results were obtained in our laboratory in which we (Sundar, S., Becker, K., & Weiss, J.) measured the effects of stressors of increasing intensity on a variety of cellular immune components. Figure 4 shows the effects of NK cell activity; the same effects were seen on T-cell mitogenesis, IL-2 production, and expression of IL-2 receptors. Figure 4 shows the effect of five different stress conditions on NK cell activity: No-stress ("No"), in which animals were simply removed from their cages for measurement; handling ("Han"), in which animals were handled for 1 min a day for 4 days; 3-shock ("3 sk"), in which the animals received 3 brief foot shocks (each 0.5 s in duration) in addition to handling; 2-hours ("2hr"), in which the animals received 2 hr of tail shock; and 19-hours ("19hr"), in which the animals received 19 hr of tail shock.

One can see that 19 hours of tail shock produced very profound suppression of NK cell activity. This is prototypical of what severely stressful conditions do not only to NK cell activity but also to a wide range of immune responses. Thus, severe stress is clearly immunosuppressive. On the other hand, one can clearly see that animals exposed to milder stress, usually the "3-shocks" condition, showed enhancement of cellular immune responses. This is indicative of the fact that a moderate degree of stress can potentiate immune responses. These two observations can be said to parallel the effects of a very strenuous exercise regimen and a moderate one, in which immunosuppression is seen with strenuous regimens and immunoenhancement with moderate ones.

In addition to the foregoing, Figure 5 shows results from a well-known study by Monjan and Collector (1976). It can be seen that an

NK ACTIVITY: SPLENOCYTES

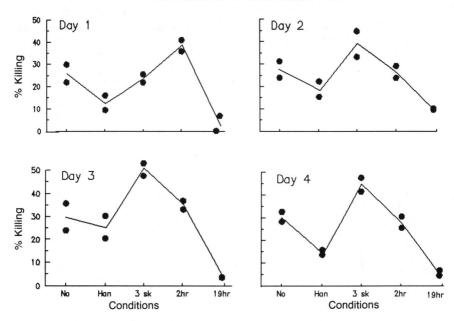

Figure 4.   Splenic natural killer-cell (NK) activity for animals of five different stressor conditions. The conditions are No (no stress), Han (handled for 4 days), 3 sk (handled plus three brief shocks), 2hr (handled plus 2 hr of tail shock), and 19hr (handled plus 19 hr of tail shock); they are placed on the abscissa in order of increasing stressfulness of the condition (left to right). The value for every animal in this study is shown, the experiment consisting of four replications (Days 1–4) with each replication containing two subjects in each of the five different conditions. Values in the figure are the percentage of target cells (YAC cells) lysed (ratio of effector:target cell is 100:1).

initially immunosuppressive stressor (exposure to noise) eventually resulted in immunoenhancement when the stressor was continued for many days. Thus, reported exposure to a stressor can produce immunoenhancement even if the initial effect is immunosuppressive. This can be seen as equivalent to the observation that exercise training, or physical conditioning, tends to ameliorate immunosuppressive effects that would occur with equivalent exercise in an untrained person and/or potentiate immunoenhancing effects. (Of course, this conclusion excludes extremely strenuous regimens of continued exercise, which are immunosuppressive.)

It is highly interesting to a stress researcher, then, that certain fundamental relationships that characterize the effects of "classical" stressors on cellular immune responses can be observed in studies of the effects of exercise on immune responses. As pointed out earlier, investigators

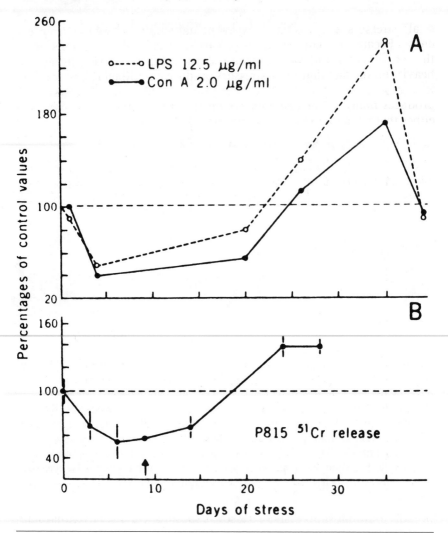

Figure 5. Stress-induced alteration of cellular immune responses as a function of number of days of exposure to the stressor. The stressor was noise. At top (A) is shown the mitogenic response of splenic lymphocytes to the mitogens LPS and Con A. At bottom (B) is shown the ability of lymphocytes to kill target cells. The mean and standard error is shown. From "Stress-Induced Modulation of the Immune Response" by A.A. Monjan and M.I. Collector, 1976, *Science*, **196**, 307–308. Copyright 1977 by the AAAS.

who are interested in exercise have often used the terms *exercise* and *stress* interchangeably, and this would have seemed a naive assumption to one familiar with stress research in general; nevertheless, several similar influences on immune responses can be seen to derive from "classical" stressors as revealed in experimental studies as well as from exercise. Because the consequences of various "classical" stressors used in the experimental studies (e.g., electric shock, restraint) apparently depend heavily on the fact that these stressors produce emotional responses (e.g., Mason, 1968a, 1968b), it is indeed intriguing to find that physical exercise produces many of the same effects on immune responses. This means either that physical exercise and emotional excitement share many of the same final common pathways to the immune system or that the effects of emotional stressors need to be considered in terms of their effects on physical activity. In any event, the commonality of some of their fundamental effects on immune responses is an intriguing observation that we hope will stimulate further research in the fields of both exercise and stress responses.

Acknowledgment

Preparation and writing of this manuscript were supported by the Behavioral Medicine Research Center of the Duke University Medical Center. The author gratefully acknowledges the valuable assistance of Sheryl Fleener in the preparation of this manuscript.

References

Brahmi, Z., Thomas, J.E., Park, M., Park, M., & Dowdeswell, I.R. (1985). The effect of acute exercise on Natural Killer-Cell activity of trained and sedentary human subjects. *Journal of Clinical Immunology,* **5,** 321–328.

Bartrop, R.W., Luckhurst, E., Lazarus, L., Kilch, L.G., & Penny, R. (1977). Depressed lymphocyte function after bereavement. *Lancet,* **1,** 834–836.

Cannon, J.G., & Dinarello, C. (1984). Interleukin-1 activity in human plasma. *Federation Proceedings* (Abst. 1034), 462.

Cohen-Cole, S., Cogen, R., Stevens, A., Kirk, K., Gaitan, E., Hain, J., & Freeman, A. (1981). Psychosocial, endocrine, and immune factors in acute necrotizing ulcerative gingivitis ("trenchmouth"). *Psychosomatic Medicine,* **43,** 91.

Eskola, J., Ruuskanen, O., Soppi, E., Viljanen, M.K., Jarvinen, M., Toivonen, H., & Kouvalainen, K. (1978). Effect of sport stress on lymphocyte transformation and antibody formation. *Clinical Experimental Immunology,* **32,** 339–345.

Fernandes, G., Rozek, M., & Troyer, D. (1986). Reduction of blood pressure and restoration of T-cell immune function in spontaneously hypertensive rats by food restriction and/or by treadmill exercise. *Journal of Hypertension,* **4**(Suppl. 3), S469–S474.

Glaser, R., Rice, J., Speicher, C.E., Stout, J.C., & Keicolt-Glaser, J.K. (1986). Stress depresses interferon production and natural killer cell activity in humans. *Behavior Neuroscience*, **100**, 675–678.

Greene, W.A., Betts, R.F., Ochitill, H.N., Iker, H.P., & Douglas, R.G., Jr. (1978). Psychosocial factors and immunity: A preliminary report (abstract). *Psychosomatic Medicine*, **40**, 87.

Horstman, D.M. (1950). Acute poliomyelitis: Relation of physical activity at the time of onset to the course of the disease. *Journal of American Medical Association*, **142**, 236.

Jemmott, J.B., III, Borysenko, J.Z., Borysenko, M., McClelland, D.C., Chapman, R., Meyer, D., & Benson, H. (1983). Academic stress, power motivation, and decrease in salivary secretory immunoglobulin A secretion rate. *Lancet*, **1**, 1400–1402.

Jensen, M.M. (1968). The influence of stress on murine leukemia virus infection. *Proceedings of the Society of Experimental Biology and Medicine*, **127**, 610–614.

Joasoo, A., & McKenzie, J.M. (1976). Stress and the immune response in rats. *International Archives of Allergy and Applied Immunology*, **50**, 659–663.

Keller, S.E., Weiss, J.M., Schleifer, S.J., Miller, N.E., & Stein, M. (1981). Suppression of immunity by stress: Effect of a graded series of stressors on lymphocytes stimulation in the rat. *Science*, **213**, 1337–1399.

Keller, S.E., Weiss, J.M., Schleifer, S.J., Miller, N.E., & Stein, M. (1983). Stress-induced suppression of immunity in adrenalectomized rats. *Science*, **221**, 1301–1304.

Kiecolt-Glaser, J.K., Garner, W., Speicher, C.E., Penn, G., & Glaser, R. (1984). Psychosocial modifiers of immunocompetence in medical students. *Psychosomatic Medicine*, **46**, 7–14.

Kiecolt-Glaser, J.K., Glaser, R., Strain, E., Stout, J., Tarr, K., Holliday, J., & Speicher, C. (1986). Modulation of cellular immunity in medical students. *Journal of Behavior Medicine*, **9**, 5–21.

Kimzey, S.L. (1975). The effects of extended spaceflight on hemotologic and immunologic systems. *Journal of American Medical Womens Association*, **30**, 218–232.

Levinson, S.O., Milzer, A., & Lewin, P. (1945). Effect of fatigue, chilling and mechanical trauma on resistance to experimental poliomyelitis. *American Journal of Hygiene*, **42**, 204.

Mason, J.W. (1968a). A review of psychoendocrine research on the pituitary-adrenal cortical system. *Psychosomatic Medicine*, **30**, 576.

Mason, J.W. (1968b). A review of psychoendocrine research on sympathetic-adrenal medullary system. *Psychosomatic Medicine*, **30**, 631.

Monjan, A.A., & Collector, M.I. (1976). Stress-induced modulation of the immune response. *Science*, **196**, 307–308.

Okimura, T., Ogawa, M., & Yamauchi, T. (1986). Stress and immune responses III. Effect of restraint stress on delayed type hypersensitivity (DTH) response, natural killer (NK) activity and phagocytosis in mice. *Japan Journal of Pharmacology*, **41**, 229–235.

Palmblad, J., Cantell, K., Strander, H., Froberg, J., Karlson, C-G., Levi, L., Granstrom, M., & Unger, P. (1976). Stressor exposure and immunological response in man: Interferon-producing capacity and phagocytosis. *Journal of Psychological Research, 20*, 193–199.

Pitkin, D.H. (1965). Effect of physiological stress on the delayed hypersensitivity reaction. *Proceedings of the Society of Experimental Biology and Medicine, 120*, 350–351.

Rasmussen, A.F., Jr., March, J.T., & Brillo, N.Q. (1957). Increased susceptibility to herpes simplex in mice subjected to avoidance-learning stress or restraint. *Proceedings of the Society of Experimental Biology and Medicine, 96*, 183–189.

Reyes, M.P., & Lerner, A.M. (1976). Interferon and neutralizing antibody in sera of exercised mice with coxsackievirus B-3 myocarditis (39204). *Proceedings of the Society for Experimental Biology and Medicine, 151*, 333–338.

Solomon, G.F. (1969). Stress and antibody responses in rats. *International Archives of Allergy, 35*, 97–104.

Targan, S., Britvan, L., & Dorey, F. (1981). Activation of human NKCC by moderate exercise: Increased frequency of NK cells with enhanced capability of effector-target lytic interactions. *Clinical Experimental Immunology, 45*, 352–360.

Viti, A., Muscettola, M., Paulesu, L., Bocci, V., & Almi, A. (1985). Effects of exercise on plasma interferon levels. *Journal of Applied Physiology, 59*, 426–428.

Watson, R.R., Moriguchi, S., Jackson, J.C., Werner, L., Wilmore, J.H., & Freund, B.J. (1985). Modification of cellular immune functions in humans by endurance exercise training during B-adrenergic blockade with atenolol or propranolol. *Medical Science in Sports Exercise, 18*, 95–100.

Weinstein, L. (1973). Poliomyelitis—a persistent problem. *New England Journal of Medicine, 288*, 370–372.

Wister, R., Jr., & Hildermann, W.H. (1960). Effects of stress on skin transplantation immunity in mice. *Science, 131*, 159–160.

Oxidants and Antioxidants and the Biological Effects of Physical Exercise

Lester Packer
University of California
Berkeley, California

Free radicals arise in vivo from environmental sources or from metabolism. It is generally agreed that they cause damage to DNA and membranes and alter gene expression, which may lead to cancer, aging, and other pathology. Oxygen-derived free radicals are stimulated by metabolism due to exercise. We seek to understand the role of oxygen-derived free radicals and their antioxidants in mechanisms of cellular injury and protection. Physical exercise in animals and humans provides an excellent model system where the interactions between oxygen radicals and antioxidants may be studied.

The generation of oxygen radicals is difficult to quantitate because of their elusive nature, due to rapid reaction. However, their presence can be inferred from changes in the level of antioxidants in the tissues or from changes in the oxidation state of antioxidants. Our new results using two model systems concern exercise-induced oxidation of glutathione (GSH) in human blood (Gohil, Viguie, Stanley, Brooks, & Packer, 1987) and changes in the level of vitamin E and ubiquionone in tissues of the rat accompanying exercise training (Gohil, Rothfuss, Lang, & Packer, 1987).

Exercise and Aging

An open and still unresolved question is whether a sustained program of physical exercise throughout life affects the pattern of human aging by changing the mean or the maximal life span. Six decades ago, Pearle (1928) advanced the Rate of Living Hypothesis, stating that increased metabolic activity was associated with acceleration of the aging process. This idea received substantial support over the last four decades from physiologists who deduced that the basal metabolic rate of 60 to 70 animal species was inversely related to the species's life span. Similarly it has

85

been shown that a life span of a species is directly correlated with the activity of superoxide dismutase (Tolmasoff, Ono, & Cutler, 1980), one of the major ubiquitous antioxidant defense enzymes present in every aerobic cell.

Direct experimental evidence for the Rate of Living Hypothesis has so far come only from studies with cold-blooded animals (poikilotherms). Two types of experiments have been pursued by many laboratories through the same course of the last three decades. First, it has been shown that varying the environmental temperatures within a certain range for several species of invertebrate insects causes changes in the rate of oxygen consumption. For example, as temperature is raised between 15 °C and 30 °C, oxygen consumption will show a more or less linear increase. Animals subjected to higher temperatures show an inverse relationship with life span (Sohal, 1984). Higher metabolic activity is associated with shorter life span. Interestingly, studies showed the same total oxygen consumption for different insect species over their life span. Even more convincing data from the invertebrate model system has come from Shaker mutants of Drosophila that have neurological alterations; these mutants have higher metabolic activity and exhibit higher oxygen consumption than the wild-type control. A plot of the life span of these species in relation to the reciprocal of the oxygen consumption activity reveals a linear relationship for the large number of Shaker mutants examined (Trout & Kaplan, 1970). Hence, studies with the invertebrate systems support the concept that increased physical activity correlates inversely with life span.

Similar experiments have been carried out in vertebrate animals. Species of salmon studied in the laboratory of Walford (Liu & Walford, 1975) exhibited longer life spans when kept at 15 °C as compared with 20 °C. The benefit of temperature on life span was exhibited mainly when the temperature was at 20 °C for 8 months and 15 °C thereafter in the later part of the life span. These authors did not conclude that the increase in life span was due to metabolic activity. Rather they chose to interpret the experiments in terms of a suppression by the lower temperature of increased autoimmune reactions that occur with aging and may shorten life span. It is still an open question for the fish model system whether decreases in swimming exercise are correlated with increase in life span due to decreased metabolic activity or for other reasons.

Comparable experiments have not been made in warm-blooded vertebrate animals or in humans, although a few isolated studies do exist. For example, Holloszy, Smith, Vining, and Adams (1985) studied free-wheeling exercise in mice. When mice were subjected to a small (5%) dietary restriction to account for the leanness of the exercising animals, a modest increase in mean life span was recorded. Brooks's laboratory (Davies, Packer, & Brooks, 1981) has shown increased cardiovascular performance in trained as compared with sedentary rats. Further studies of this type seem necessary.

Increased oxygen consumption is known to increase the rate of oxygen radical production and to change the cellular antioxidant mechanisms. Basson, Terblanche, and Oelofsen (1982) showed that sustained exercise training of rats over many months led to increased accumulation of fluorescent damage products in muscle and other tissues compared with sedentary controls. These data indicate that increased free radical reactions occur as a result of training, but they do not clarify their importance with respect to health, aging, and longevity. It is important to obtain quantitative information about the effects of exercise on the occurrence of free radical reactions and how cellular antioxidant defenses respond to them. Are they able to cope with the damaging reactions that may be brought about by an oxygen radical cascade induced by acute exercise, even in trained individuals?

Indicators of Damage Accompanying Exercise

Many studies have shown the extent of damage to skeletal muscle and peripheral tissues that accompanies exercise. Three of the major membranes of skeletal muscle appear to incur damage by acute exercise, for example, and damage to the sarcolemma is inferred by the release into the blood of enzymes normally found in the muscle, such as lactate dehydrogenase, pyruvate kinase, and myoglobin (Schwane, Johnson, Vandenakker, & Armstrong, 1983). Mitochondrial damage is indicated by loss of respiratory control, decreases in coupling of energy synthesis to oxygen consumption, and increases in lipid peroxidation. Such changes are seen in mitochondria isolated from skeletal muscle of exercised as compared to sedentary animals (Davies, Quintanilha, Brooks, & Packer, 1982). Damage to lysosomes is indicated by the loss of a latency of enzymes. In addition, cytochemical data support enhanced lysosomal activity, particularly in the postexercise recovery period, where such activity peaks 3 days after a bout of exercise (Salminen, 1985). Lower levels of vitamin E (Aikawa, Quintanilha, Delumen, Brooks, & Packer, 1984; Gohil, Viguie et al., 1987) and changes in glutathione oxidation in skeletal muscle (Lew, Pyke, & Quintanilha, 1985) are indicative of the occurrence of free radical reactions. Increased levels of stable free radicals (ESR signals) have been noted after exercise in animals (Davies et al., 1982).

In peripheral tissues and erythrocytes, changes in osmotic fragility have been noted, as have changes in the ratio of reduced to oxidized glutathione. Increased mitochondrial damage, decreased lysosomal latency, increased lipid peroxidation and stable free radicals, and changes in the ratio of reduced to oxidized glutathione are some indices that suggest oxidative stress in the liver following exercise (Davies et al., 1982). Massive accumulation of erythrocytes and hemoglobin in fecal material is attributed to damage to the ileum. Loss of iron occurs as a result of damage to the ileum and also is attributed to loss of myoglobin and hemoglobin through kidney excretion. This contributes to the iron depletion that accompanies "runner's anemia" (Hunding, Jordal, & Paulev, 1981; McCord, 1985; Packer, 1986).

Repair of Damage

It seems clear that much of the damage described reverts to normal in the postexercise recovery period. Delayed-onset soreness, which peaks at about 3 days, is a harbinger of the repair process following a severe bout of damaging exercise (Schwane et al., 1983). During this period, leukocytes invade the damaged tissues and participate in repair processes (Schaefer, Kokot, Heidland, & Plass, 1987).

Repetitive bouts of exercise result in adaptive changes. Muscle tissues display the well-known increased biogenesis of mitochondria, changes in fiber types, and increased levels of antioxidant enzymes (Quintanilha & Packer, 1983). Nevertheless, even trained individuals display postexercise indices of damage and repair after a bout of strenuous exercise. The unanswered question is whether there are any long-term cumulative effects as a consequence of a regular program of training.

Exercise and Aging: Speculations on the Trade-Offs

The improvement in cardiovascular performance with exercise training is generally believed to have a positive effect on mean life span. In addition, trained individuals tend to be lean, and there is a correlation between high dietary fat intake, decreased cardiovascular performance, and increased cancer risk. Aging is also affected by leanness, as dietary or caloric restriction extends the life span (Holeman & Merry, 1986; Masoro, 1985; Weindruch, Walford, Sligiel, & Guthrie, 1986).

Dietary or caloric restriction, as contrasted with malnutrition, represents a classical experiment in gerontology. Many species of invertebrates and vertebrates have been shown to display marked increases in mean and total life span when grown under dietary restriction throughout their life (Holeman & Merry, 1986; Masoro, 1985). Many ideas have been considered as the underlying causes that allow dietary-restricted animals to experience such marked life span extensions, including effects on the endocrine system and the immune system (decreased autoimmunity) among others. One interesting recent observation is the finding that dietary-restricted animals display an increase in one of the major enzymes involved in hydroperoxide removal (catalase) and a decrease in lipid peroxidation of liver tissue (Koizumi, Weindruch, & Walford, 1987). Thus, an exercise program during aging could possibly result in positive benefits on mean life span.

On the other hand, exercise increases the generation of free radicals and the accumulation of damage products such as fluorescent damage product (lipofuscin). Oxidative damage to proteins (Oliver, Ahn, Moerman, Goldstein, & Stadtman, 1987) and nucleic acid constituents also occur. With repetitive bouts of exercise, this may result in changes in physiological parameters and pathology. Cumulative effects and effects on critical cellular systems are not well known, although it is suspected that the damage may change the death pattern. Although cardiovascular-related disorders diminish, cancer and kidney failures increase.

It is important to design a more comprehensive experiment that will optimize diet and dietary restriction, antioxidant status, and programs of exercise to demonstrate whether mean and total life spans are altered by a regular program of physical exercise. The expense and difficulty of undertaking experiments of this type may now be overcome.

Such experiments may provide new insights into the merits of various hypotheses for aging. The Rate of Living Hypothesis (Pearl, 1928) and the Free Radical Hypothesis (Harman, 1981) could be tested more rigorously. Consideration of the Autoimmune Hypothesis (Weindruch et al., 1986) and the Error Catastrophe Hypothesis (i.e., the relative balance between genetic and environmental factors in the aging process) may enable us to reformulate more comprehensive hypotheses about the biological effects of exercise, including the underlying events surrounding the generation of free radicals and protection by antioxidants to modulate various physiological and pathological responses in the body. Investigating the stress of exercise may be extremely valuable in evolving newer understandings of the relationship between physical activity, human well-being, and aging.

References

Aikawa, K.M., Quintanilha, A.T., Delumen, B.O. Brooks, G.A., & Packer, L. (1984). Exercise endurance training alters vitamin tissue levels and red cell hemolysis in rodents. *Bioscience Reports, 4,* 253–257.

Basson, A.B.K., Terblanche, S.E., & Oelofsen, W. (1982). A comparative study of the effects of aging and training on the levels of lypofuscin in various tissues of the rat. *Comparative Biochemistry and Physiology, 71A,* 369–374.

Davies, K.J.A., Packer, L., & Brooks, G.A. (1981). Biochemical adaptations of mitochondria, muscle, and whole animal respiration to endurance training. *Archives of Biochemistry & Biophysics, 109,* 538–553.

Davies, K.J.A., Quintanilha, A.T., Brooks, G.A., & Packer, L. (1982). Free radicals and tissue damage produced by exercise. *Biochemical and Biophysical Research Communications, 107,* 1198–1205.

Gohil, K., Viguie, C., Stanley, W.C., Brooks, G.A., & Packer, L. (1987). Blood glutathione oxidation during human exercise. *Journal of Applied Physiology, 64,* 115–119.

Gohil, K., Rothfuss, L., Lang, J., & Packer, L. (1987). Effect of exercise training on tissue, vitamin E and ubiquinone content. *Journal of Applied Physiology, 63,* 1638–1641.

Harman, D. (1981). The aging process. *Proceedings of the National Academy of Sciences, 78,* 7124–7128.

Holeman, A.M., & Merry, B.J. (1986). The experimental manipulation of aging by diet. *Biological Reviews, 61,* 329–368.

Holloszy, J.O., Smith, E.K., Vining, M., & Adams, S. (1985). Effect of voluntary exercise on longevity of rats. *Journal of Applied Physiology, 59,* 826–831.

Hunding, A., Jordal, R., & Paulev, P.E. (1981). Runners anemia, an iron deficiency. *Acta Medica Scandinavica, 109,* 315–318.

Koizumi, A., Weindruch, R., & Walford, R.L. (1987). Influences of dietary restriction and age on liver enzyme activities and lipid peroxidation in mice. *Journal of Nutrition, 117,* 361–367.

Lew, H., Pyke, S., & Quintanilha, A. (1985). Changes in the glutathione status of plasma, liver, and muscle following exhaustive exercise in rats. *Federation European Biochemical Societies Letters, 185,* 262–266.

Liu, R.K., & Walford, R.L. (1975). Mid life temperature transfer effects on life span of annual fish. *Journal of Gerontology, 30,* 129–131.

Masoro, E.J. (1985). Nutrition and aging—a current assessment. *Journal of Nutrition, 115,* 842–848.

McCord, J. (1985). Oxygen-derived free radicals in postischemic tissue injury. *New England Journal of Medicine, 312,* 159–163.

Oliver, C.N., Ahn, B-W., Moerman, E.J., Goldstein, S., & Stadtman, E.R. (1987). Age-related changes in oxidized protein. *Journal of Biological Chemistry, 262,* 5488–5491.

Packer, L. (1986). Oxygen radicals and antioxidants in endurance exercise. In G. Benzi, L. Packer, & N. Siliprandi (Eds.), *Biochemical Aspects of Physical Exercise* (pp. 73–92). New York: Elsevier.

Pearl, R. (1928). *The Rate of Living.* New York: Knopf.

Quintanilha, A.T., & Packer, T. (1983). Vitamin E, physical exercise and tissue oxidative damage. In *Ciba Foundation Symposium 101 on Biology of Vitamin E* (pp. 56–69). London: Pitman Press.

Salminen, A. (1985). Lysosomal changes in skeletal muscles during the repair of exercise injuries in muscle fibres. *Acta Physiologica Scandinavica, 124*(Suppl. 539).

Schaefer, R.M., Kokot, K., Heidland, A., & Plass, R. (1987). Jogger's leucocytes. *New England Journal of Medicine, 316,* 223–224.

Schwane, J.A., Johnson, S.R., Vandenakker, & Armstrong, R.B. (1983). Delayed-onset muscular soreness and plasma CPK and LDH activities after downhill running. *Medicine and Science in Sports and Exercise, 15,* 51–56.

Sohal, R.S. (1984). Metabolic rate, free radicals and aging in free radicals. In D. Armstrong, R.S. Sohal, R.G. Cutler, & T.F. Slater (Eds.), *Molecular Biology, Aging, and Disease* (pp. 119–127). New York: Raven Press.

Tolmasoff, J.M., Ono, T., & Cutler, R. (1980). Superoxide dismutase: Correlation with life span and specific metabolic rate in primary species. *Proceedings of the National Academy of Sciences, 77,* 2777–2781.

Trout, W.E., & Kaplan, W.D. (1970). A relation between longevity, metabolic rate, and activity in Shaker mutants of drosophila melanogaster. *Experimental Gerontology, 5,* 83–92.

Weindruch, R., Walford, R.L., Sligiel, S., & Guthrie, D. (1986). Retardation of aging in mice by diet restriction: Longevity, cancer, immunity and life time energy intake. *Journal of Nutrition, 116,* 641–654.

Physical Activity as a Stimulus to Changes in Gene Expression in Skeletal Muscle

Frank W. Booth
The University of Texas Medical School
Houston, Texas

An exciting era is upon us wherein exercise scientists will be able to employ techniques of molecular biology to gain new insights into the mechanisms by which skeletal muscle adapts to a new phenotype because of physical training. This review identifies several research questions in this area that might be regarded as the most important for work over the next decade. Five potential research areas—protein translation, gene transcription, growth factors, protein function, and gene regulation—were selected for review as the important focus points for future research into the mechanisms by which physical activity alters gene expression in skeletal muscle. Most of these approaches could be applied to any tissue, cell type, or protein that adapts to repeated bouts of daily exercise (physical training).

Protein Translation

From the studies reported in the literature to date, acute changes in protein synthesis rate in fast-twitch skeletal muscle during or immediately after an exercise bout in the first few days of training seem usually to be under translational control, which is defined as regulation of binding of a messenger ribonucleic acid (mRNA) to the 80S ribosome. On the other hand, after a period of 2 to 8 days of physical training, changes in mRNA levels occur. Because it is unknown whether these increases in mRNA are due to either an increase in its synthesis or a decrease in its degradation, the increase in mRNA levels after a few days of training is designated as a change in pretranslational control.

I give here some of the evidence supporting the hypothesis that translational control plays an important role in determining rates of protein synthesis in fast-twitch skeletal muscles in the first few hours after altering muscle usage. If fast-twitch muscle is electrically stimulated for 10 min

91

in a perfused hemicorpus preparation, protein synthesis is decreased to zero within minutes of the start of exercise and then returns to normal levels within minutes of ending the electrical stimulation (Bylund-Fellineus, Ojama, Flaim, Li, Wassner, & Jefferson, 1984). Messenger RNA could not have changed this rapidly. During the electrical stimulation of rabbit fast-twitch muscle for 12 hr/day, it took to the 10th day of stimulation to observe an increase in citrate synthase mRNA, whereas the activity of citrate synthase had already increased by the 2nd stimulation day (Seedorf, Leberer, Kirschbaum, & Pette, 1986). These reports imply a translational control of protein synthesis for fast-twitch muscle during acute exercise.

We have noted that decreases in the synthesis rates of specific proteins, such as cytochrome c and actin, occur prior (in the time scale of days) to decreases in their mRNA concentrations in atrophying fast-twitch muscles of immobilized limbs (Morrison, Montgomery, Wong, & Booth, 1987; Watson, Stein, & Booth, 1984). Furthermore, we have observed that the percentage change from control values for cytochrome c synthesis rates and actin synthesis rates in recovering atrophied fast-twitch muscle after ending limb immobilization parallels changes in corresponding mRNA levels for the first 2 days of recovery (Morrison, Muller, & Booth, 1987; Morrison et al., 1987). By the fourth recovery day the percentage increases in cytochrome c and actin synthesis rates exceeded the percentage increases in their mRNAs, which infers regulation of their protein synthesis rates by both pretranslational and translational controls.

However, the literature is not completely one-sided. There are examples where a change in a protein level appears to be due exclusively to a change in pretranslational control, without any alteration of translational control. For example, the declines in parvalbumin protein and parvalbumin mRNA paralleled one another during a 20-day period of 12 hr/day electrical stimulation (Leberer, Seedorf, & Pette, 1986). Another exception to the apparent role of translational control in acute exercise is the observation that certain types of regulatory molecules are induced rapidly by transcriptional control. For example, Izumo, Isomyama, Nadal-Ginard, and Mahdavi (1987) found that within 3 hr after pressure overload of the rat heart, the mRNAs encoding c-*fos*, c-*myc* and heat shock protein hsp 70 were induced to very high levels. They suggested that the increase in these mRNAs reflects early changes in the nuclei of myocardial cells. A similar observation has been made by Komuro, Kurabayaski, and Takaku (1987), who found increases in c-*fos* mRNA and c-*myc* mRNA in the heart 2.5 hr after aortic constriction was started. These observations suggest that at a time when translational control is altering the synthetic rates of mitochondrial and contractile proteins in skeletal muscle during acute exercise, there may be a simultaneous change in the transcriptional control of mRNAs for proteins thought to regulate growth.

Few if any studies have been performed to delineate how the mechanisms controlling translation are altered by an acute change in the quantity of muscle contraction. Part of the reason is that the techniques to perform such measurements have only recently been developed and are sometimes difficult to perform and to interpret. An impetus to the development of techniques to study mechanisms controlling translation is the information that translational control of protein synthesis plays an important role in the dramatic switch that occurs from cellular to viral protein synthesis after adenovirus or influenza virus infection. These studies by oncologists are advancing methodologies to research translational control. A future area of research for exercise physiologists will be to delineate the molecular pathways by which an acute change in exercise level results in translational control of protein synthesis by the application of certain procedures from oncology and other fields.

Numerous cofactors determine the rate of translation (Moldave, 1985; Pain, 1986). Guanine nucleotide exchange factor (GEF) facilitates the displacement of guanosine diphosphate (GDP) from eukaryotic initiation factor 2 (eIF-2) and its replacement by guanosine triphosphate (GTP). Recently Jefferson and Kimball (1988) reported that the impairment in peptide-chain initiation in fast-twitch skeletal muscle of diabetic rats is related to a decrease in GEF activity. An increase in the phosphorylation status of eIF-2 would cause GEF activity to decrease. Other modes to alter the translation efficiency have been described. Secondary and tertiary folding of liver ferritin mRNA is suggested to be necessary for the binding of a repressor of translation of the mRNA (Wang, Dickey, & Theil, 1988).

Gene Transcription

It is now well established that certain types of chronic exercise will lead to a change in the level of an mRNA in skeletal muscle. An inconclusive list of examples is given here. Williams and coworkers (Williams, Salmons, Newsholme, Kaufman, & Mellor, 1986; Williams, Garcia-Moll, Mellor, Salmons, & Harlan, 1987) have reported the following: increases in mitochondrial protein mRNAs in the rabbit tibialis anterior muscle after 10 and 21 days of continuous electrical stimulation; F_1-ATPase β-subunit mRNA (2.2- and 2.3-fold after 10 and 21 days, respectively); cytochrome oxidase VIC-subunit mRNA (1.3- and 1.9-fold); and cytochrome b (not determined and 5-fold). These increases paralleled increases in mitochondrial enzyme capacities. In the same studies Williams et al. (1986) observed increases in the enzymatic capacity of citrate synthase (2.1- and 5.5-fold) and cytochrome oxidase (2.1- and 4.1-fold) after 10 and 21 days, respectively, of continuous electrical stimulation. Decreases in mRNA levels and protein levels have been noted in atrophying skeletal muscles. We (Morrison, Montgomery, Wong, & Booth, 1987; Morrison, Muller, & Booth, 1987) noted a 53% decrease in cytochrome c mRNA and a 41% decrease in cytochrome c protein per muscle after 7 days of limb immobilization of the red quadriceps, which caused a 22% loss in muscle wet weight. Likewise, Morrison, Muller, & Booth observed a 61% decrease in α-actin mRNA per gastrocnemius-plantaris muscle and an approximate 27% loss in actin per muscle after 7 days of limb immobilization. Thus, after 7 to 21 days of altered muscle usage, the direction of the change in the amount of a specific mRNA parallels the directional change in the content of its protein in skeletal muscle.

The next logical question could be, What are the molecular signal(s) for the change in mRNA level by exercise? The first step to answer this question is to determine which of the following occur: an increase in gene transcription, a more efficient processing of the immature heterogeneous nuclear RNA into mature mRNA, an increased stability of the mRNA in the sarcoplasm, or a combination of these that causes increased mRNA quantities during physical training. The inference that the increased gene transcription is the cause of the increased mRNA quantity for exercised skeletal muscles has not been proven.

In the future it will be necessary to prove directly that increased exercise results in an increased transcription rate of an mRNA from a gene. (I argue in the gene regulation section of this review that obtaining an answer that is closest to the truth about exercise effects on a specific gene's transcription rate requires usage of an identical exercise protocol in a whole animal model as the exercise protocol performed in humans. Such an argument requires using adult animals). The methodology available at present to estimate gene transcription is identified as nuclear runoff or transcriptional runoff assay. However, application of this technique to adult skeletal muscle has limitations. The first limitation of a nuclear runoff assay is that the isolated nuclei from adult skeletal muscle of animals are impure and have low yields with published techniques. Regarding the impurity problem, the likelihood of preferential recovery of myonuclei and fibronuclei from adult skeletal muscle between control and exercise groups has not been experimentally addressed.

It is known that exercise disrupts connective tissue in skeletal muscle (Jones, Newham, Obletter, & Giamberardino, 1987), which may activate fibroblast mitotic activity. Such changes in connective tissue could cause a preferential recovery, but this speculation must be tested. A second limitation, of possibly greater importance, is the fact that within experimental groups variability for transcriptional runoffs is so high that the treatment must cause a difference greater than twofold in order to obtain statistical significance. Many types of human exercise, such as lifting a weight 24 times a day for a total of 1 minute of load bearing or running 30 min a day, may not be of sufficient intensity to produce an increase greater than twofold in transcriptional rate.

Although inferential reasoning could imply that transcription rates of genes must have been altered to permit the conversion of a fast-twitch muscle to a slow-twitch muscle during the continuous chronic stimulation of a skeletal muscle, such logic cannot substitute for direct measurements. Inferential reasoning is applied to the following example: When fiber types are converted from slow- to fast-twitch by removal of the weight-bearing function of the soleus muscle, myosin isoforms previously not expressed appear (Thomason, Herrick, Surdyka, & Baldwin, 1987; Thomason, Herrick, & Baldwin, 1987). From such an observation it is feasible to hypothesize that the most logical way for a new protein to be expressed is for its mRNA, which previously was absent, to appear. Alternatively it could be argued that prior to the treatment, a heterogeneous nuclear RNA was transcribed, but it was immediately degraded so that no mRNA could be detected. In the latter case it could be logically suggested that the removal of weight bearing by hind-limb suspension could result in an increased stability of this mRNA, so that it appeared in the sarcoplasm and was translated. To determine with greater certainty what the truth is, future studies in exercise physiology should document directly whether transcription increases in nuclei.

At present there are techniques available to identify *cis* control regions of genes and to isolate *trans* factors that interact with *cis* control regions. A *cis* control region is a specific DNA sequence, which is usually upstream of the gene that regulates, in part, the transcription of the gene. Deletion of a positive *cis* regulatory DNA sequence in a mutant construct of the gene, in which all other normal sequences are present, causes a decreased transcription of the gene. The presence of a *cis* sequence alone is not usually sufficient for transcription of a gene. Factor(s) must interact with *cis* sequences. These factors are either proteins or oligonucleotides and are called *trans* factors because they are not a part of the DNA molecule upon which they act. At this time it is fair to hypothesize that an alteration in exercise level by skeletal muscle leads to a cascade of second messengers that culminate in either the appearance or the disappearance of a *trans* factor, which could be called an exercise *trans* factor. The appearance of an exercise *trans* factor could interact with a *cis* region of a gene, upregulating its transcription.

On the other hand, the disappearance of a *trans* factor because of exercise could remove its presence at a *cis* site, repressing gene transcription. It is known that many adaptations to exercise training consist of parallel changes in the quantities of numerous proteins (Green, Reichmann, & Pette, 1983; Holloszy, Oscai, Don, & Mole, 1970). A possible explanation for the coordinate control of a subset of muscle genes to exercise training could be explained by exercise's production of a common *trans* factor which interacted with identical *cis* regions found upstream of each of the genes from the subset. This idea has experimental support. Comparisons with the upstream regulatory regions of known muscle gene sequences revealed homologies for a 17-nucleotide element in the muscle creatine kinase gene, α skeletal actin gene, and myosin heavy chain gene (Jaynes, Chamberlain, Buskin, Johnson, & Hauschka, 1986).

Although all of the identification of *cis* regulatory regions within the DNA sequences for genes could be done in cultured muscle cells, there is a major potential limitation of extrapolating from muscle culture identified *trans* factors to exercise adaptations in vivo. It has been reported that the relative importance between two regulatory *cis* regions of a certain gene to the gene's transcription was dependent on the type of transformed muscle cells used in tissue culture (Muscat & Kedes, 1987). When DNA sequences between -626 and -1300 nucleotides upstream of the TATA box (a conserved adenine-thymine rich septamer found about 25 bases before the startpoint of each eukaryotic RNA polymerase II transcription unit) of the human α-actin gene were removed and the mutant construct was then transfected (placed) into C2C12 myotubes, 93% of the transcriptional activity of the human α-actin gene was lost. However, transfection of the same mutant into L8 myotubes resulted in only a 20%

loss in transcriptional activity. To reduce transcriptional activity of the human α-actin gene in the L8 myotubes to the low levels of C2C12 myotubes, the nucleotides -87 to -626 had to be removed from the actin mutant in L8 myotubes. Muscat & Kedes interpreted their data to infer that different *trans* factors were present in the two types of skeletal muscle cultures. One or more *trans* factors, which interacted with DNA sequences that were -626 to -1300 base positions before the TATA box of the human α-actin gene, were present in the sarcoplasm of C2C12 myotubes, but not in the L8 myotubes. We infer from this interpretation that identification of in vivo exercise *trans* factors may not be made with 100% certainty in immortalized muscle cultures because in the process of their transformation certain normal cellular expressions, such as *trans* factors, were altered in the C2C12 and L8 muscle cell lines.

How do you prove with 100% certainty that transformation of a muscle cell does not eliminate any of its exercise *trans* factors? (Other limitations to muscle culture—such as the failure to produce the gravity effect on muscle in vivo and the failure to obtain expression of adult protein isoforms—are discussed elsewhere in this review.) A possible mode to circumvent the described limitations in the identification of "exercise" *trans* factors would be to couple the procedure of in vivo footprinting (Jackson & Felsenfeld, 1987) with the isolation of potential *trans* factors by their attachment to an immobilized oligonucleotide, which is of identical DNA sequence to the *cis* DNA sequence that was footprinted.

Growth Factors

In the past, exercise physiologists have concentrated their search for exercise-induced growth signals on the area of alterations in blood hormone levels. Unfortunately, no role for an exercise-induced change in blood hormone concentration has been documented to be the causal factor either for the increase in mitochondrial density during endurance training or for the increase in muscle size during load training. For example, the increase in mitochondrial enzyme concentration during the one-leg training by humans only occurred in the trained leg, but there was no change in the nontrained leg (Morgan, Cobb, Short, Ross, & Gunn, 1971). Such an observation questions a primary role for the change in the level of a blood hormone inducing mitochondrial biogenesis. Exercise-induced hypertrophy of skeletal muscle has been produced in many animal models of hormone deficiency (Goldberg, Etlinger, Goldspink, & Jablecki, 1975). All of these studies infer that exercise training produces a local signal within the exercising muscle that elicits the adaptation in muscle protein.

Numerous polypeptide growth factors have been shown to affect myoblast differentiation in cultured muscle cells (Florini, 1987). Insulin-like growth factor I enhances cell proliferation and stimulates myoblasts to form postmitotic myotubes in cultured muscle cells (see Florini for references). Insulin-like growth factor I also likely stimulates growth of adult skeletal muscle (Turner, Rotwein, Novakofski, & Bechtel, 1988). Fibroblast growth factor stimulates proliferation of cultured muscle cells and represses muscle differentiation (Clegg & Hauschka, 1987). Transforming growth factor-β is a potent inhibitor of myoblast differentiation in several cultured cell lines (Ewton, Spizz, Olson, & Florini, 1988). Thus it is possible that polypeptide growth factors induced by exercise could have a paracrine action to alter gene expression.

Some of the retroviral research done in recent years has accelerated the identification of autocrine growth factors. A widely held hypothesis is that retroviruses have captured truncated portions of mammalian genes that encode either for autocrine growth factors or for components of signal pathways for growth, such as cell-surface receptors, cytoplasmic guanine nucleotide-binding proteins, and protein kinases (Pawson, 1987). For example, v-*sis* oncogene is a truncated portion of platelet-derived growth factor, the v-*ras* family of oncogenes are derived from G-proteins, and v-*erb* A oncogene is a fragment of the thyroid hormone receptor and is homologous to the family of steroid hormone-binding receptor genes. Whereas mammalian genes involved in growth are controlled, expression of retroviral oncogenes upon their integration into the host genome is not regulated. The continuous production of proteins from oncogene mRNAs in the infected mammalian cells is thought to induce unrestrained proliferation as each oncogene mimics a different step in signal pathways for cellular growth or for cellular proliferation. The significance of these observations in virology to the field of exercise physiology is that behavioral patterns of oncogenic proteins might provide templates for experiments to identify autocrine, or local, growth factors induced in normal muscle cells by exercises such as weight bearing.

A recent example of how identification of oncogenes leads to information about control of transcription in normal cells was given by Pawson (1987). A novel oncogene, v-*jun* (viral-*jun*) was found and sequenced. Upon comparison of the sequence of v-*jun* to all known sequences in a computer bank, its 91 terminal residues were found to be very similar to two other known DNA sequences. One of these homologous sequences was to a DNA-binding domain which, when a yeast *trans* factor called GCN4 was bound, activated a DNA enhancer that caused the increased transcription of a family of genes required for amino acid synthesis. The other sequence homologous to the v-*jun* that was found in the computer search was a DNA sequence found in normal mammalian DNA; it was designated c-*jun* (cellular *jun*). (Earlier in this review I stated that retroviral species captured a portion of mammalian DNA into the retrovirus' DNA. The viral gene is designated v-*jun* whereas the normal cellular gene is called c-*jun*). Because the protein made by c-*jun* in normal cells was not known, a computerized comparison of the amino acid sequence of GCN4 (the *trans* factor that bound to a region of yeast DNA homologous to v-*jun*) to all known amino sequences for proteins was performed; and a protein similar to GCN4 was found.

This protein, AP-1, is a known *trans* factor that binds to the enhancer elements of numerous genes, such as SV-40, metallothionein IIA and collagenase. Because all of these genes are induced by phorbol esters, Pawson (1987) postulates that activation of protein kinase C by phorbol esters could phosphorylate AP-1, activating the *trans* factor so that it could interact with gene enhancer regions. The information described (see Pawson) could serve as a template for future exercise research. Is it possible that identification of a retroviral oncogene causing unregulated proliferation of muscle cells would lead to the identification of a cellular protein in normal cells that mediates signal transduction from weight lifting to increased expression of a family of contractile proteins? In the future, identification of retroviruses causing rhabdomyoblastomas might provide clues to the identity of normal growth factors in normal muscles.

Protein Function

The glucose transporter is an example of a protein for which the application of molecular biological techniques to genetically engineer mutant glucose transporters in C2C12 muscle cells might assist in delineating mechanisms by which exercise alters glucose uptake. First, background information about glucose uptake by exercising skeletal muscle will be summarized briefly, and then potential ideas on how a mutant glucose transporter protein could assist in delineating a postexercise mechanism will be given. A recent hypothesis stated by Young, Uhl, Cartee and Holloszy (1986) is that when glucose uptake into muscle is accelerated to replenish depleted glycogen stores postexercise, the rapid glucose uptake results in a greater rate of glucose transporter cycling back to its intracellular storage site or to a greater rate of glucose transporter degradation. The consequence, according to Young et al., would be a lower steady state level of glucose transporters in the sarcolemma and a reversal of the exercise-induced activation of glucose transport.

Some of the information that is available to construct mutant glucose transporters could be applied to planning experiments to test the hypothesis of Young et al. (1986) as to how exercise alters glucose uptake. The complete amino acid sequence of the glucose transporter from a human hepatoma cell has been deduced from the nucleotide sequence of a cDNA clone by Mueckler et al. (1985). From the deduced sequence they proposed that the protein crosses the sarcolemma 12 times in the form of hydrophobic α helices. With domain-specific antibodies, Davies, Meeran, Cairns, and Baldwin (1987) showed that the C-terminal domain of the glucose transporter bound cytochalasin β and was in the cytoplasm. It has already been hypothesized (Shows et al., 1987) that variants of the glucose transporter in non-insulin dependent diabetes mellitus (NIDDM) patients could constitute a class of postreceptor defects that contribute to their hyperglycemia. Application of such a hypothesis to exercise physiology leads to the suggestion to engineer genetically a glucose transport mutant that could not bind glucose, or alternatively that would not insert into the sarcolemma, and then to monitor both glucose uptake and compartmentalization of the glucose transporter postexercise.

Levels of glucose transporter mRNAs have already been monitored in various tissues. In transformed hepatocytes, which have an enhanced glucose uptake, increased glucose transporter mRNA was noted (Flier,

Mueckler, McCall, & Lodish, 1987). A hypothesis in oncology is that the increased glucose metabolism by the tumor initiates a feedback to up-regulate levels of glucose transporter mRNA. Using this hypothesis, an additional hypothesis could be generated that endurance types of training would cause an increased glucose transporter mRNA and glucose transporter protein. Experiments such as the following could be performed to test the hypothesis. Can the training effect on skeletal muscle for glucose uptake be mimicked by transfection of a glucose transporter gene with a regulatory sequence that has been engineered to be continuously activated so that high levels of glucose transporter mRNA are expressed in C2C12 muscle culture? What happens to muscle glycogen levels in these cells? The potential to answer many questions about how exercise modulates glucose uptake into skeletal muscle, or in fact any exercise-modulated protein, might be answered with molecular biological techniques such as those described with other procedures not mentioned here.

Gene Regulation

The principal method for identifying those DNA sequences that regulate the transcription of a specific gene is first to delete, or mutagenize, a small segment of DNA sequences that are usually just before the start of contiguous sequences that provide the code for an mRNA and second to test whether the mutated DNA fragment results in altered transcription of the gene after its introduction into cells (Dynan & Tjian, 1985). If an eliminated segment of DNA from the gene causes reduction of its transcription, then the segment may play a role in the up-regulation of transcription of gene. These techniques are now in wide use (Maniatis, Goodbourn, & Fischer, 1987), mostly in cultured cells rather than in vivo.

At this stage of research development in exercise physiology, it is appropriate to ask whether a valid approximation of the identification of those DNA sequences that modulate or regulate gene transcription in vivo in response to exercise training can be achieved in tissue culture or whether whole animals should be studied. It is my bias that exclusive use of muscle cells in culture will not always provide the true identity of *cis* regulatory regions of genes modulating exercise-induced changes in protein levels, nor will they always provide the correct identification of *trans* factors whose levels and interactions with gene regulatory regions are altered by exercise. If certainty of the validity of tissue culture experiments is in doubt, then in vivo approaches will be necessary to confirm or deny the tissue culture results. So, why do both, and why not just start with the in vivo model? The following paragraphs provide the possible limitations of using cultures of muscle cells to evaluate gene transcription for studies on the mechanisms by which, for example, weight lifting or daily running alter the gene expression in a skeletal muscle.

One limitation to muscle cells in culture in exercise physiology research is the inability in tissue culture to mimic human exercise programs. For example, chronic tension that is imposed on muscle when it supports the body against gravity is thought to play a major role in the maintenance of muscle mass and of muscle tension capacity (Alford, Roy, Hodgson, & Edgerton, 1987; Winiarski, Roy, Alford, Chiang, & Edgerton, 1987). For muscle cells in culture to undergo contraction against gravity, they would have to contract under a load. To date, muscle cells have been stretched unloaded in tissue culture (Vandenburgh, 1987). However, the quality of gene expression by a muscle likely differs between an unloaded stretched muscle and a muscle that contracts against a load while being stretched. Muscles that are stretched unloaded in vivo have longer muscle fibers with no change in fiber diameter (Spector, Simard, Fournier, Sternlicht, & Edgerton, 1982), whereas muscles contracting under a load in vivo (as in weight lifting) have increased fiber diameter with minimal increase in fiber length. Thus adaptations in protein quantities after physical training that occur in vivo cannot always be reproduced in cultures of muscle cells. This conclusion infers that different *trans* factors would be induced by exercise in vivo from those produced by mimicking exercise in cultured muscle cells. If different *trans* factors are produced, this implies that different *cis* regions on DNA would be protected in footprinting experiments.

A second limitation to the use of cultured muscle cells to study exercise-induced gene adaptations is that transformed cells express embryonic, not adult, protein isoforms. For example, embryonic muscle cells express embryonic myosin heavy chain, but not adult fast or slow myosin heavy chain (Mahdavi, Strehler, Periasamy, Wieczorek, Izumo, & Nadal-Ginard, 1986). Thus cultured immortalized cell lines cannot be used to investigate how limb suspension (removal of weight bearing by the hind limbs of rats) causes the down-regulation of adult slow myosin heavy chain protein (Thomason, Herrick, Surdyka, & Baldwin, 1887; Thomason, Herrick, & Baldwin, 1987).

Thus transformed muscle cell lines may not always provide a valid approximation of the true changes in *trans* factors and of true DNA regulatory regions through which an exercise-initiated signal changes gene transcription in the whole animal. If the *trans* factors that are expressed in muscle cell cultures as a result of mimicked exercise are different from those actually evoked in vivo by more appropriate exercise regimens, the following question can be raised: How do we determine which experiment using exercised muscle cells in culture gives the true *trans* factor change seen in vivo, and which culture experiment does not provide the correct *trans* factor induced by exercise in vivo? If the ideas previously expressed are true, it seems logical that the course of action most likely to produce less effort over the long term and to provide information closer to the truth is to identify *cis* regulatory regions of genes activated by the "exercise" *trans* factor(s) induced in whole animals. The alternative course of action would be first to perform experiments in tissue culture that undergoes "exercise" and then to repeat the same experiments in vivo to determine which tissue culture experiments were valid and which provided incorrect "exercise" *trans* factors and thus incorrect *cis* identifications.

In vivo footprinting is a technique that can be used to accurately map the sites of sequence-specific protein–nucleic acid interactions ("footprints") in the whole animal (Jackson & Felsenfeld, 1987). Once the nucleic acid sequence of the protein-binding region has been identified by in vivo footprinting, a synthetic oligonucleotide of identical sequence to this region can be synthesized and used in affinity chromatography to analyze nuclear sap. Proteins that bind to the oligonucleotide would be candidates for *trans* factors interacting with the *cis* region in vivo.

Another common technique in molecular biology that is used for determination of regulatory regions of genes is the transfection of mutant recombinants into cells in tissue culture. The mutant recombinant could consist of a constituent-regulated enhancer-promotor region attached to the mutated gene for the glucose transporter protein. (As suggested earlier, regions required for the exercise response of the glucose transporter protein can be delineated in tissue culture.) The mutant recombinant could consist also of a mutant regulatory region of a muscle-specific gene attached to a recorder gene such as chloramphenicol acetyltransferase.

Summary

The research questions I chose to address were selected from a coalescence of the current techniques available in the fields of molecular biology and cell biology to the current knowledge in the exercise physiology area that researches mechanisms of change in gene expression by physical training.

Because of the length limitation of this review, some potential areas of research into training-induced mechanisms, such as transduction of exercise-initiated signals through existing second-messenger systems, could not be covered here. This limitation can be viewed positively because it implies that the future holds more exciting questions about the mechanisms of exercise-induced gene expression in skeletal muscle than can be suggested in a short review. One of the major questions to be answered in the future is, How do each of the individual mechanisms by which molecules, muscle fibers, whole muscles, and other organs integrate so that a live, unanesthetized animal is able to adapt to repeated exercise and consequently to work with less fatigue after training? The field of exercise physiology is embarking on a new frontier where ultimately it will be possible to explain how the human adapts to environmental perturbations.

Acknowledgments

Stimulating discussions with Dr. Thomason and Mr. Wong assisted in the formation of certain ideas. Mr. Wong also assisted in editing the review. The manuscript was typed by Ms. Stefanie Duhon. Grant AR 19393 supported this work. This article is dedicated to Dr. Robert Haubrich upon his retirement as professor of biology at Denison University. As my advisor he initiated the present review in 1965 when he asked in an oral exam how I would alter the genetic makeup to make a world-class athlete.

References

Alford, E.K., Roy, R.R., Hodgson, J.A., & Edgerton, V.R. (1987). Electromyography of rat soleus, medial gastrocnemius, and tibialis anterior during hind limb suspension. *Experimental Neurology*, **96**, 635-649.

Bylund-Fellineus, A.-C., Ojama, K.M., Flaim, K.E., Li, J.B., Wassner, S.J., & Jefferson, L.S. (1984). Protein synthesis versus energy state in contracting muscles of perfused rat hindlimb. *American Journal of Physiology*, **246**, E297-E305.

Clegg, C.H., & Hauschka, S.D. (1987). Heterokaryon analysis of muscle differentiation: Regulation of the postmitotic state. *Journal of Cell Biology*, **105**, 937-947.

Davies, A., Meeran, K., Cairns, M.T., & Baldwin, S.A. (1987). Peptide-specific antibodies as probes of the orientation of the glucose transporter in the human erythrocyte membrane. *Journal of Biological Chemistry*, **262**, 9347-9352.

Dynan, W.S., & Tjian, R. (1985). Control of eukaryotic messenger RNA synthesis by sequence-specific DNA-binding proteins. *Nature*, **316**, 774-778.

Ewton, D.Z., Spizz, G., Olson, E.N., & Florini, J.R. (1988). Decrease in transforming growth factor -β binding and action during differentiation in muscle cells. *Journal of Biological Chemistry*, **263**, 4029-4032.

Flier, J.S., Mueckler, M., McCall, A.L., & Lodish, H.F. (1987). Distribution of glucose transporter messenger RNA transcripts in tissues of rat and man. *Journal of Clinical Investigation*, **79**, 657-661.

Florini, J.R. (1987). Hormonal control of muscle growth. *Muscle & Nerve*, **10**, 577-598.

Goldberg, A.L., Etlinger, J.D., Goldspink, D.F., & Jablecki, C. (1975). Mechanism of work-induced hypertrophy of skeletal muscle. *Medicine and Science in Sports*, **7**, 248-261.

Green, H.J., Reichmann, H., & Pette, D. (1983). Fibre type specific transformations in the enzyme activity pattern of rat vastus lateralis muscle by prolonged endurance training. *Pflugers Archives*, **399**, 216-222.

Holloszy, J.O., Oscai, L.B., Don, I.J., & Mole, P.A. (1970). Mitochondrial citric acid cycle and related enzymes: Adaptive response to exercise. *Biochemical and Biophysical Research Communications*, **40**, 1368-1373.

Izumo, S., Isomyama, S., Nadal-Ginard, B., & Mahdavi, V. (1987). Acute pressure overload causes rapid induction of the proto-oncogenes and a stress protein gene in the myocardium. *Circulation*, **76**(Suppl. 4), 477.

Jackson, P.D., & Felsenfeld, G. (1987). *In vivo* footprinting of specific protein-DNA interactions. In S.L. Berger & A.R. Kimmel (Eds.), *Guide to Molecular Cloning Techniques* (pp. 735-755). Orlando: Academic.

Jackson, P.D., & Felsenfeld, G. (1987). *In vivo* footprinting of specific protein-DNA interactions. *Methods in Enzymology*, **152**, 735-755.

Jaynes, J.B., Chamberlain, J.S., Buskin, J.N., Johnson, J.E., & Hauschka,

S.D. (1986). Transcriptional regulation of muscle creatine kinase gene and regulated expression in transfected mouse myoblasts. *Molecular and Cellular Biology, 6,* 2855–2864.

Jefferson, L.S., & Kimball, S.R. (1988). Regulation of peptide-chain initiation by insulin in skeletal muscle and heart. *FASEB Journal 2,* A778.

Jones, D.A., Newham, D.J., Obletter, G., & Giamberardino, M.A. (1987). Nature of exercise-induced muscle pain. *Advances in Pain Research Therapy, 10,* 207–218.

Komuro, I., Kurabayashi, M., & Takaku, F. (1987). Expression of cellular oncogenes during development and pressure-overload hypertrophy of the rat heart. *Circulation, 76*(Suppl. 4), 476.

Leberer, E., Seedorf, U., & Pette, D. (1986). Neural control of gene expression in skeletal muscle. Calcium-sequestering proteins in developing and chronically stimulated rabbit muscles. *Biochemical Journal, 239,* 295–300.

Mahdavi, V., Strehler, E.E., Periasamy, M., Wieczorek, D.F., Izumo, S., & Nadal-Ginard, B. (1986). Sarcomeric myosin heavy chain gene family: Organization and pattern of expression. *Medicine and Science in Sports and Exercise, 18,* 299–308.

Maniatis, T., Goodbourn, S., & Fischer, J.A. (1987). Regulation of inducible and tissue-specific gene expression. *Science, 236,* 1237–1245.

Moldave, K. (1985). Eukaryotic protein synthesis. *Annual Review of Biochemistry, 54,* 1109–1149.

Morgan, T.E., Cobb, L.A., Short, F.A., Ross, R., & Gunn, D.R. (1971). Effects of long-term exercise on human muscle mitochondria. *Advances in Experimental Medicine and Biology, 11,* 87–95.

Morrison, P.R., Montgomery, J.A., Wong, T.S., & Booth, F.W. (1987). Cytochrome c protein synthesis rates and mRNA levels during atrophy and recovery in skeletal muscle. *Biochemical Journal, 241,* 257–263.

Morrison, P.R., Muller, G.W., & Booth, F.W. (1987). Actin synthesis rate and mRNA level increase during early recovery of atrophied muscle. *American Journal of Physiology, 253,* C205–C209.

Mueckler, M., Caruso, C., Baldwin, S.A., Panico, M., Blench, I., Morris, H.R., Lienhard, G.E., Allard, W.J., & Lodish, H.F. (1985). Sequence and structure of a human glucose transporter. *Science, 229,* 941–945.

Muscat, G.O., & Kedes, L. (1987). Multiple 5'-flanking regions of the human α-skeletal actin gene synergistically modulate muscle-specific expression. *Molecular and Cellular Biology, 7,* 4089–4099.

Pain, V.M. (1986). Initiation of protein synthesis in mammalian cells. *Biochemical Journal, 235,* 625–637.

Pawson, T. (1987). Transcription factors as oncogenes. *Trends in Genetics, 3,* 333–334.

Seedorf, U., Leberer, E., Kirschbaum, B.J., & Pette, D. (1986). Neural control of gene expression in skeletal muscle. Effects of chronic stimulation on lactate dehydrogenase isoenzymes and citrate synthase. *Biochemical Journal, 239,* 115–120.

Shows, T.B., Eddy, R.L., Byers, M.G., Fukushima, Y., deHaven, C.R., Murray, J.C., & Bell, G.I. (1987). Polymorphic human glucose transporter gene (GLUT) is on chromosome 1 p. 31.3 p. 35. *Diabetes,* **36,** 546–549.

Spector, S.A., Simard, C.P., Fournier, M., Sternlicht, E., & Edgerton, V.R. (1982). Architectural alterations of rat hind-limb skeletal muscles immobilized at different lengths. *Experimental Neurology,* **76,** 94–110.

Thomason, D.B., Herrick, R.E., Surdyka, D., & Baldwin, K.M. (1987). Time course of soleus muscle myosin expression during hindlimb suspension. *Journal of Applied Physiology,* **63,** 130–137.

Thomason, D.B., Herrick, R.E., & Baldwin, K.M. (1987). Activity influences on soleus muscle myosin during rodent hindlimb suspension. *Journal of Applied Physiology,* **63,** 138–144.

Turner, J., Rotwein, P., Novakofski, J., & Bechtel, P. (1988). Induction of mRNA for IGF-1 and -II during growth hormone stimulated muscle hypertrophy. *American Journal of Physiology,* **255,** E513–E517.

Vandenburgh, H.H. (1987). Motion into mass: How does tension stimulate muscle growth? *Medicine and Science in Sports and Exercise,* **19,** S142–S149.

Wang, Y.-H., Dickey, L.F., & Theil, E.C. (1988). The importance of untranslated regions of ferritin mRNA in translational control. *FASEB, Journal,* **2,** A778.

Watson, P.A., Stein, J.P., & Booth, F.W. (1984). Changes in actin synthesis and α-actin-mRNA content in rat muscle during immobilization. *American Journal of Physiology,* **247,** C39–C44.

Williams, R.S., Salmons, S., Newsholme, E.A., Kaufman, R.E., & Mellor, J. (1986). Regulation of nuclear and mitochondrial gene expression by contractile activity in skeletal muscle. *Journal of Biological Chemistry,* **261,** 376–380.

Williams, R.S., Garcia-Moll, M., Mellor, J., Salmons, S., & Harlan, W. (1987). Adaptation of skeletal muscle to increased contractile activity. *Journal of Biological Chemistry,* **262,** 2764–2767.

Winiarski, A.M., Roy, R.R., Alford, E.K., Chiang, P.C., & Edgerton, V.R. (1987). Mechanical properties of rat skeletal muscle after hind limb suspension. *Experimental Neurology,* **96,** 650–660.

Young, D.A., Uhl, J.J., Cartee, G.D., & Holloszy, J.O. (1986). Activation of glucose transport in muscle by prolonged exposure to insulin. Effects of glucose and insulin concentrations. *Journal of Biological Chemistry,* **261,** 16049–16053.

A Discussion of the Scientific Presentations

R. Sanders Williams
Duke University Medical Center
Durham, North Carolina

In an effort to introduce a high degree of critical analysis into this conference, each scientific presentation of the first day was reviewed by an independent investigator with special expertise in a specific area of medicine or biology pertinent to the topic under discussion (e.g., lipoprotein or glucose metabolism). In order to maintain the broad and critical perspective that was the goal of the conference, most reviewers were selected from among scientists who do not routinely pursue studies of the effects of physical activity per se, but who are recognized as experts within their respective fields. These critiques served as the focus for a general discussion that is summarized briefly in the following paragraphs.

Cardiovascular Adaptations to Physical Activity

In the discussion of the presentation by Saltin, Mitchell pointed out the somewhat surprising discrepancy between measurements of maximal oxygen consumption in athletes and their performances in track events. Saltin reiterated the important concept that maximal oxygen consumption should be viewed as a predictor of the maximal rate at which work can be performed, whereas other factors determine the length of time that work can be sustained. Maximal oxygen consumption is limited primarily by the pump capacity of the heart, whereas endurance time is influenced heavily by metabolic features (e.g., mitochondrial content and glycogen concentrations) of the skeletal muscles. Most programs of physical training induce adaptations in both cardiac performance and the oxidative capacity of the trained skeletal muscles, so that maximal oxygen consumption and endurance capacity tend to be highly correlated. However, these variables can be dissociated rather dramatically during detraining, when adaptive responses of skeletal muscles to a previous training regimen are reversed more rapidly than cardiovascular adaptations, and endurance times decline much more rapidly than maximum oxygen consumption.

Williams commented that endurance performance may be a more clinically relevant measurement than maximal oxygen consumption in patients with cardiovascular diseases and that this distinction is often overlooked in studies that evaluate the efficacy of drugs or other measures used for the treatment of angina pectoris or congestive heart failure. Saltin also emphasized that maximum oxygen consumption can be altered by only 30% to 50% as a function of training, whereas endurance performance can be increased by 200% to 400%.

Hormonal Adaptations to Physical Activity

Blackshear responded to the presentation by Richter and focused on two features of the effects of physical activity on endocrine systems as important areas for future research. The possibility that amenorrhea induced by exercise training may be associated with osteoporosis is of considerable concern, and the interrelationships between caloric intake, exercise habits, and sex hormone release and metabolism should be clarified.

More information is also needed to define more fully the role of physical activity in the therapy and prevention of Type II diabetes. Blackshear cited data that 80% to 90% of persons affected by Type II diabetes in this country are inadequately controlled, and effective measures to prevent microvascular and macrovascular complications of this disease are urgently needed. Current recommendations of the American Diabetes Association identify exercise as a useful adjunct to diet and pharmacologic therapy of Type II diabetes, but note that most of the evidence that supports the efficacy of physical training in ameliorating this condition is based on studies performed in animals and in normal humans. Additional studies of the effects of habitual activity on insulin sensitivity of peripheral tissues, on pancreatic β-cell responsiveness to hyperglycemia, and on the clinical course of patients with Type II diabetes are required. Richter noted that, in the limited studies that have been performed in patients, physical activity produced favorable effects on insulin sensitivity and glycosylated hemoglobin concentrations, but that these effects have been disappointingly small. Furthermore, the effects of physical activity on insulin sensitivity in humans are quite short-lived and may last only for a few days following cessation of exercise.

In further discussion of Type II diabetes, Richter employed an analogy to drug therapy to emphasize that the short-lived nature of the effects of physical activity on glucose metabolism need not detract from its potential clinical utility, because physically active individuals tend to exercise almost daily. However, the transient nature of the effects of exercise on insulin sensitivity must be considered in the design of human investigations. As a final point, all discussants agreed that habitual exercise may be more important in preventing the onset of Type II diabetes in genetically susceptible individuals than in reversing the disease once it has become established.

Effects of Physical Activity on Lipoprotein Metabolism

Dunn led the discussion of the presentation by Wood. In considering the utility of habitual exercise in the treatment of hyperlipidemias, Dunn noted that considerable physical activity (8 to 12 miles of jogging for several months) appears to be required to produce major effects. Furthermore, Dunn noted the more striking effects of physical activity in elevating HDL-C than in lowering LDL-C and emphasized that the hypothesis that raising plasma concentrations of HDL-C will reduce the risk of cardiovascular disease is less supported than the corresponding hypothesis concerning the reduction of LDL-C. He also identified three research questions of special interest: elucidation of the interrelationships between exercise, diet, and body composition as determinants of plasma concentrations of lipoproteins; clarification of the mechanisms by which physical activity promotes an increase in HDL-C; and analysis of the effects of physical activity on LDL receptors.

Wood agreed that direct evidence was stronger for a favorable effect on cardiovascular risk of lowering LDL-C than for the benefits of raising HDL-C. However, he emphasized the powerful inverse relationship between HDL-C and coronary risk in epidemiologic studies. In addition, he pointed out that the major clinical trials that have documented the benefits of pharmacologic therapy to lower LDL-C have been performed at tremendous cost, and similar resources have not been (and are not likely to be) expended to examine effects of raising HDL-C. Wallace pointed out the greater difficulty in effecting changes in HDL-C than in LDL-C in patient populations, but Wood responded that, in addition to exercise training, several newer hypolipidemic drugs promote increases in HDL-C as well as decreases in LDL-C. Wood also stated that future research concerning physical activity and lipoprotein metabolism should examine subfractions of LDL and HDL.

Effects of Exercise on Biological Features of Aging

The discussion of Shephard's remarks was led by Cohen and raised several interesting questions of both practical and theoretical significance. Cohen first commented that, although examination of the effects of physical activity in aged populations has focused primarily on maximal oxygen consumption and other measurements of peak cardiovascular performance, other variables may be of greater clinical importance. Physical characteristics such as ankle stability, abdominal muscle strength, and balance are taken for granted in younger individuals, but may be major determinants of the capacity of older persons to live independently. Cohen and Shephard agreed that these latter variables, as well as cardiovascular performance, may be amenable to change by physical activity.

Cohen focused upon the striking diversity that is observed when almost any physiological variable is measured in elderly individuals to advance the concept of "successful" versus "usual" aging. The existence of certain elderly individuals who have favorable characteristics (successful aging) suggests that many of the deleterious characteristics attributed to the aging process are not inevitable and that a worthwhile and potentially attainable goal would be to convert the "usual" pattern to the "successful" one.

Wallace expressed the opinion that research designed to clarify the effects of physical activity on aging appeared to be hindered by the absence of a working definition of aging as a biological process and by a failure to distinguish the intrinsic rate of aging from the rate of accrual of disease events. Cohen was supported by Fridovich in the viewpoint that there is a genetically determined maximum life span for each species, including humans. However, the effects of many external factors are superimposed on this intrinsic process. Among these external factors, some are subject to modification (e.g., diet and physical activity), while others are beyond the control of the individual. This concept of aging therefore identifies at least three tiers of factors (genetically determined intrinsic aging, uncontrollable external factors, and controllable external factors) that affect the state of the organism at any given age, even in the absence of disease events.

Effects of Exercise and Other Forms of Stress on Immunological Competence

Haynes responded to the presentation by Weiss. Studies of the effects of the AIDS virus indicate that the immune system has a phenomenal reserve. In the normal state it functions at a high level, and it is likely that any intervention designed to improve immune competence will, at best, produce effects that are subtle. On the other hand, insults to the immune system that produce major deleterious effects can have catastrophic consequences. Thus, in clinical studies, deleterious effects of stresses such as unaccustomed exhaustive exercise or overtraining must be major before one would expect to detect clinical manifestations of an impairment of the immune system, and it is unlikely that clinically significant enhancement of immunological competence from physical conditioning can be detected in short-term studies.

Following these caveats, Haynes discussed possible approaches to answer the following question: Can we condition the immune system to make it work better? He noted that progress in basic immunology will provide tools suitable for examination of subtle changes and will make this task easier. He singled out studies of lymphokines as an example of this progress and cited data from clinical studies of patients with autoimmune diseases such as rheumatoid arthritis and lupus erythematosis. In patients with these diseases, viral infections are uncommon during periods in which the underlying disease is active. When patients go into remission, gamma interferon levels (which are high during periods of active disease) fall, and herpes virus infections are common. In addition, minor variations in immune function may take on more importance in elderly persons, and interventions that produce only subtle effects on immunologic competence may have greater clinical relevance in this population.

Returning to the question of stress-induced suppression of immune function, Wallace asked Stray-Gundersen, physician to the U.S. Olympic cross-country ski team, to comment on the susceptibility of these athletes to infection. Stray-Gundersen replied that viral infections were extraordinarily frequent during periods of intense training. At these times endurance athletes have low absolute lymphocyte counts, low salivary IgA, and high plasma levels of cortisol. In addition, their susceptibility to respiratory infections is probably increased from the dessicating effects of moving high volumes of cold, dry air across the respiratory mucosa during training, from the dry air encountered during prolonged and frequent air travel, and from exposure at national and international competitive events to individuals harboring diverse viruses. Weiss commented that competitive athletes may be particularly valuable as experimental subjects for stress research because they voluntarily subject themselves to stress situations that are both chronic and severe.

Physiological Significance of Free Radicals Generated During Exercise

Fridovich responded to the presentation by Packer. He first added evidence in support of the hypothesis that free radicals are involved in processes that determine longevity. He stated that the rate of urinary excretion of thymine glycol, a metabolite produced during repair of DNA damaged by free radical-induced hydroxylation of nucleotide bases, suggests that humans experience this mechanism of DNA damage at least 1,000 times daily. Furthermore, when species of different life spans are compared, there is an inverse relationship between longevity and the rate of thymine glycol excretion. Fridovich cautioned against extrapolation of data from studies of oxidative injury and longevity in insects to higher organisms, because the cells of insects undergo terminal differentiation as they become adults and insect tissues do not undergo the constant remodeling characteristic of most mammalian tissues.

There was considerable discussion of the evidence that physical activity is associated with accelerated generation of free radicals in skeletal muscle and whether this process is in fact associated with tissue damage in skeletal muscle or in other tissues. In his presentation Packer had described human studies demonstrating increased oxidation of glutathione in erythrocytes and an increased content of lipofuscin in muscle following exhaustive exercise. Fridovich questioned the validity of extrapolating results in erythrocytes to muscle and the specificity of the lipofuscin data. He also stated that increased flux through the electron transport chain, which clearly occurs in exercising muscles, is not obligatorily linked to increased production of free radicals. He suggested the experiment of measuring exhalation of pentane, a volatile end product of oxidation of polyunsaturated fatty acids by free radicals, prior to and following exercise in humans.

Packer replied that pentane excretion is increased twofold following exercise in human subjects and correlates inversely with plasma concentrations of the antioxidant vitamin E. He reiterated that evidence for tissue damage by free radicals generated during exercise was based largely on methods that are indirect and imprecise, but maintained that the evidence is nevertheless quite persuasive. In animal studies glutathione oxidation occurs in many tissues, not just erythrocytes; electron spin resonance studies provide direct evidence for free radical generation; lipid peroxidation products are produced; and membrane damage following exhaustive exercise is evident by the appearance of cytoplasmic muscle proteins in plasma. He speculated that delayed onset muscle soreness and ileal mucosal damage following extreme exercise may be clinical manifestations of free radical-induced membrane damage.

Williams asked for an explanation of potential mechanisms by which free radicals generated within skeletal muscle could induce tissue damage in remote tissues. Fridovich replied that repair of membranes containing lipid peroxides can result in generation of lipid hydroperoxides, which circulate in blood and have the potential to cause damage to remote tissues.

Dohm commented that it is probably important to distinguish between unaccustomed or exhaustive exercise and less extreme exercise. Only the former types of exertion are associated with muscle soreness or release of muscle enzymes. Dohm also stated that there is no evidence of a higher incidence of cancer in physically active individuals, suggesting that DNA damage by free radicals is not appreciably increased by regular exercise.

Physical Activity as a Stimulus to Changes in Gene Expression in Skeletal Muscle

Williams selected two aspects of the presentation by Booth for special emphasis. Unlike some of the other biological effects of habitual physical activity discussed at this conference, the changes in mitochondrial content and oxidative capacity of skeletal muscles produced by endurance training are large, reproducible, and of unequivocal physiological significance. Furthermore, the underlying biology of this adaptive response has been characterized extensively in terms of muscle ultrastructure and protein biochemistry. These features suggest that efforts to understand the molecular biology of mechanisms by which physical activity results in adaptations in biological systems should begin with studies of this response in skeletal muscle.

Emerging techniques for analysis of mechanisms of gene regulation provide powerful tools that may make this task feasible in the next few years. However, a major problem that has hindered this effort so far is the absence of a suitable cell culture model. Skeletal myotubes from avian and mammalian sources can readily be grown in culture and can be induced to contract in a tonic manner for days. However, under the culture conditions that have been analyzed so far, contractile activity of cultured myotubes does not result in adaptations in mitochondrial enzymes similar to those that are induced by endurance training of skeletal muscles in situ. The apparently different effects of tonic contractile activity on intact muscles of adult animals and on cultured myotubes may reflect only technical inadequacies of the artificial culture environment (e.g., mechanical disruption of cell membranes during vigorous contractions) that can be overcome in future experiments. On the other hand, more fundamental biological differences (e.g., immaturity of cultured myotubes, paracrine effects of endothelial cells or neurons) may preclude entirely the development of a cell culture model of endurance training for molecular biological investigations.

Even in the absence of a cell culture model, the effects of contractile activity on gene regulation in skeletal muscles may be studied productively by in vitro analyses of intact muscles from whole animals and perhaps by studies of heterologous promoters in transgenic animals subjected to training regimens.

In a discussion of animal models currently used for studies of gene regulation by contractile activity in muscle, Williams and Booth concurred that unphysiological models, such as continuous electrical stimulation of the motor nerve, are useful for this purpose. However, Booth emphasized that one should not assume that mechanisms of gene regulation in such extreme models will be identical to those involved in adaptive responses to endurance training.

Concluding Remarks

Haskell concluded the discussion session and selected a single point for renewed emphasis. In considering the potential health benefits of habitual physical activity we must be aware that biological effects of exercise have a dose-response relationship and a biological half-life. Certain desirable effects of exercise may be induced with only short durations of low intensity (low dose) exercise, whereas other effects will become manifest only after prolonged and/or intense (high dose) exercise. The biological half-life of certain desirable effects of exercise may extend for many days following the last training session, but other effects may be limited to a period of hours following a bout of exercise. These relationships must be considered in the design of clinical studies and in efforts to advise the public about the benefits and risks of exercise. By analogy to pharmacologic therapy, the transient nature of certain biological effects of exercise (e.g., increased insulin sensitivity) does not preclude a potentially important role for exercise in the therapy or prevention of widely prevalent disease states such as Type II diabetes, hypertension, and coronary heart disease.

Part II

Major Frontiers of Exercise Research

Exercise as a Means of Maximizing Human Physical Performance and Productivity

William L. Haskell

Stanford University School of Medicine
Palo Alto, California

To perform optimally on the job and in their personal lives, persons must have *mens sana in corpore sano*—a sound mind in a sound body. How this condition is best achieved and maintained in response to the diverse goals one strives to obtain throughout life will continue to be one of the most demanding and exciting challenges to science. First, the human is intrinsically a highly complex organism, and a complete understanding of human biologic functioning is still in the distant future and will require for its elucidation more advanced technologies than exist today. As demanding as this research will be, even more difficult will be achieving a definitive understanding of human mental attributes, including how people think, learn, and remember. Along the way, it also will be necessary to establish which functions and behaviors are determined more by heredity than environment and vice versa, the causes for the substantial interindividual variation in human response to various environmental stimuli, and what modalities can be most effectively used to assist persons in maximizing performance and productivity within their genetic potential. One small aspect of this last issue is the primary focus of this presentation: what we know about the role of exercise in enhancing human physical performance and productivity.

An inspection of human anatomy and physiology makes it obvious that the human being was designed for exercise. For example, as much as 45% of human body mass is skeletal muscle, the capacity for producing energy with this large muscle mass is high, the cardiorespiratory system can support a wide range of energy expenditure for extended periods, the substrate needed for rapid energy production is available in every skeletal muscle cell in addition to a store of substrate to support moderate intensity exercise for days, and the anatomical arrangement of the musculoskeletal system allows for a diverse pattern of movements. Also, very impressive in this design is the exquisite integration by the neurohormonal system of the numerous organs and tissues that directly participate in or support body movement. It has been apparent for some time that,

115

as a result of this design, the human body functions best when it is provided with frequent opportunities to exercise: "Lack of activity destroys the good condition of every human being, while movement and methodical physical exercise save and preserve it" (Plato, 380 B.C.)

The availability of two pathways for energy production (aerobic and anaerobic) and muscle cells with two different contractile properties (fast vs. slow twitch), the capacity of the vascular system to supply and remove substances to the contracting muscle cell, and the close neurohormonal control of these functions during muscle contraction enable humans to effectively perform activities requiring a wide range of energy production (Table 1). During dynamic, rhythmic exercise using large muscle groups, such as during running, cycling, or Nordic skiing, international class sprinters can expend energy for several seconds at a rate that is greater than 35 times their rate of energy expenditure at rest, or more than 45 cal/min (sprinting at 40 kph or 25 mph). On the other hand, top-flight endurance athletes can maintain exercise for up to 2 hr that requires close to 20 times their resting energy expenditure or 24 cal/min. A good example of such a performance is running a marathon race in 2 hr and 10 min (a speed of 20 kph or 12 mph).

Heredity Versus Training

Differences in exercise capacity among individuals are due to variations in their genetic endowment, gender, and age and in their exercise training,

Table 1   Human Capacity for Energy Production During Large-Muscle, Dynamic Exercise

Activity	METS[a]	ATP (mole/min)	Calories /min[b]	$\dot{V}O_2$ ml/kg/min[c]
Sitting	1	.06	1.25	3.5
Walk @ 3 mph	3	.19	3.75	10.5
Jog @ 6 mph	10	.65	12.50	35
Run @ 10 mph	16	1.05	20.0	56
Run @ 12 mph (marathon = 2:10)	19	1.23	24.0	66
Run @ 15 mph (mile = 4 min)	24	1.57	30.0	84
Sprint @ 20 mph (100 yds = 10.2 sec)	32	2.09	40.0	112
Sprint @ 25 mph (50 yds = 4.1 sec)	38	2.48	47.5	133

[a]Multiples of resting energy expenditure. [b]Body weight of 70 kg (154 lbs).
[c]Oxygen uptake—milliliters per kilogram of body weight per minute.

nutritional, and health status. It is well established that many of the interindividual differences in exercise capacity measured in healthy adults are the result of a hereditary basis for oxygen transport capacity of the cardiovascular system, skeletal muscle metabolic capacity, and skeletal muscle mass and composition as defined by muscle fiber type (Bouchard, 1986). These genetically determined factors establish a person's absolute capacity for performance and are major determinants as to whether or not a person will be an international champion in an athletic event in which success is dominated by speed, strength, power, or endurance. The trainability of an individual also appears to have a significant genetic component (Bouchard, 1988). Much less is known about the genetic acquisition of manual skill or dexterity; thus, the role heredity plays in the success achieved in skill-dominated athletic, leisure-time, or job-related activities is not well established. However, we all know of people for whom some skill-based activities "just come naturally."

The expression of a high capacity for exercise performance usually occurs by the time a person has completed puberty or shortly thereafter and can be determined with moderate accuracy by performance tests (speed, power, strength, endurance) or by tests of biologic function or structure (VO_2max, muscle fiber typing, body composition analysis). Such testing is purported to be used in Eastern European countries to select athletes at young ages to prepare them for national teams. This process tends to happen de facto quite frequently whenever there are substantial opportunities for athletic competition at an early age. Youths with outstanding "natural attributes" tend to be successful quite rapidly at a local level and, with proper coaching and training, go on to become national or international champions. It is now very rare in the United States for top flight athletes not to have demonstrated their prowess by the time they are 20 years of age, and most do so by the time they reach age 17 (Smith, Ogilvie, Haskell, & Gaillard, 1978).

The genetically based variations in functional capacity among the general population do not play a significant role in most people's day-to-day performance or productivity, except in athletes who desire to compete on top-flight teams or to perform professionally or in individuals who inherit a trait that reduces their functional capacity to a level substantially below the norm. Much more important in determining how effectively persons meet the challenges of daily living is what they have done with the raw materials provided by their parents. Physical performance capacity, job productivity, and general quality of living are all significantly influenced by what and how much a person eats; the use of tobacco, alcohol, and recreational drugs; exposure to infectious diseases, especially in the 1980s, sexually transmitted diseases; exposure to environmental pollution or toxins; and the nature of one's habitual exercise.

Exercise to Enhance Physical Performance

Exercise can enhance physical performance or productivity by its direct effect on a person's capacity to produce energy and thus to have greater speed, strength, power, or endurance. This effect is very evident in training for athletic events like track and field, where major changes in performance can be achieved in a single season or year. At the other end of the performance spectrum are the large increases in functional capacity achieved with the exercise conditioning of patients or healthy persons who have been bed rested for several weeks or more. There should be no dispute about the potential for exercise training to increase physical performance capacity in all ambulatory individuals, except maybe for those athletes who by years of training have reached their genetically determined limits. Numerous studies have been published demonstrating significant increases in the endurance (Pollock, 1973) and strength (Atha, 1981) of males and females ages 6 to 80 years, and these changes can be achieved in most patients, including those with cardiovascular disease, diabetes, chronic obstructive pulmonary disease, arthritis, and renal failure (Skinner, 1987).

The body adapts to an increase in exercise as it does to any other stress: It responds by attempting to increase its capacity to better accommodate the biologic or physical alterations produced by the stress. For example, during endurance-type exercise, a sustained stress or demand is placed on a variety of tissues or biochemical processes, and they respond by increasing their ability to support a higher intensity of activity for the same time or the same intensity of activity for a longer period. The characteristics of the increase in activity needed to produce specific changes in functional capacity have been extensively investigated and have resulted in frequently quoted guidelines or a "pharmacopoeia of exercise," with much of the emphasis placed on endurance training.

The increase in aerobic power as measured by maximal oxygen uptake ($\dot{V}O_2$max) has been used as a general index or standard for determining the effectiveness of various exercise regimens designed to increase endurance capacity. The magnitude of the increase in $\dot{V}O_2$max with training varies with age; initial value; the exercise type and intensity; and session duration, frequency, and number. Increases in $\dot{V}O_2$max with endurance exercise training regimens consisting of brisk walking, jogging, running, cycling, or swimming, with sessions lasting for 20 to 45 min performed three to five times per week for 8 to 52 weeks, have usually ranged from 5% to 35% (Pollock, 1973). Generally the increase in $\dot{V}O_2$ max is greater the more vigorous the training up to an intensity of approximately 85% of aerobic power, the longer the training sessions up to 60 min, the more frequent the sessions up to five times per week, and the longer the training program up to 1 year (Pollock, 1973). When usual activity has been restricted during the weeks or months prior to initiating training, there is a greater increase in $\dot{V}O_2$max, with increases exceeding 50% in some cases (Saltin, Blomqvist, Mitchell, Johnson, Wildenthal, & Chapman, 1968).

For individuals interested in performing moderate to vigorous intensity exercise, it is easy to provide a regimen that will significantly increase their aerobic power within 3 months. More difficult is the recommendation to the individual who wants to exercise as little as possible but still get significant benefit. Frequently these people are told that they need to exercise three times per week for at least 20 min per session at 60% to 75% of their aerobic capacity or 70% to 85% of their maximal heart rate. These recommendations are based primarily on short-term studies, most using younger men as subjects (Pollock, 1973). Several more recent studies have found that endurance exercise training carried out at 45% to 50% of aerobic power is sufficient to significantly increase $\dot{V}O_2$ max in sedentary men and women (Gaesser & Rich, 1984; Gossard et al., 1986). For most individuals over age 40 this intensity of exercise requires no more than brisk walking.

As the population of the United States ages, it will become even more important to document what performance and health benefits can be achieved using lower intensity exercise. Also, it recently has been demonstrated that instead of exercising continuously for 30 min, a significant increase in aerobic capacity can be achieved by moderate intensity exercise performed in 10-min bouts three times per day (DeBusk, Hakanssan, Sheehan, & Haskell, 1988). More research is needed to define what other types of exercise profiles increase aerobic power or other performance- and health-related measures. What are the benefits if moderate intensity exercise is performed in six bouts of 5 min each per day rather than in one bout of 30 min? Answers to this type of question will be needed to maximize the public's participation in exercise.

The increase in aerobic power and endurance capacity can be very substantial with more vigorous, longer-term training, and it results in people being able to perform physical tasks that would have been impossible prior to training. Middle-aged men who could not jog continuously at 10 kph (6 mph) for more than 12 min prior to exercise training were able to run 10 km in less than 50 min after 1 year of moderate intensity training three to four times per week that consisted of jogging or running approximately 4 mi per session (Wood, Terry, & Haskell, 1985). Sedentary men who took up a brisk walking program (approximately 4.5 mph) for 20 weeks, 4 days per week, 40 min per session, decreased the time it took them to walk 1 mile from 12.9 to 11.1 min, a 17% increase in speed (Pollock, Miller, Janeway, Linnerud, Robertson, & Valentino, 1971).

Even in those studies where the training-induced increase in $\dot{V}O_2$ max is as much as 30%, the magnitude of this increase does not result in the weekend athlete's achieving the capacity demonstrated by successful endurance athletes. Presented in Figure 1 are representative $\dot{V}O_2$max values for men whose activity status ranges from bedrest to very active, including values for highly trained endurance athletes. Also plotted are the changes in $\dot{V}O_2$max reported from selected exercise training studies in men ranging in age from 18 to 74 years. The duration of the training programs was 12 to 52 weeks. A man with an average $\dot{V}O_2$max of 35 ml of oxygen per kilogram of body weight per minute would have to increase his aerobic capacity by at least 75% in order to achieve the capacity of most endurance athletes. These data support a major role for heredity in determining maximal aerobic power.

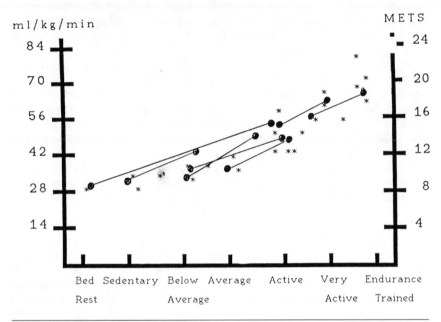

Figure 1. Maximal oxygen uptake in young healthy men. Individual symbols are the mean value from selected studies published in the literature. The symbols that are connected are training studies in healthy young men demonstrating the change in mean V̇O₂max when going from one activity classification to another. Training studies include those lasting from 16 to 26 weeks.

Enhancing Productivity by Preventing Disability

Much more at issue than the role of exercise in directly improving physical performance capacity is the nature and magnitude of the effect of exercise on productivity by its potential preventive or therapeutic benefits for major chronic degenerative disorders, especially ischemic heart disease, stroke, hypertension, adult-onset diabetes, osteoporosis, and psychologic dysfunction. Because these disorders are very prevalent in our society and can decrease functional capacity to a level that impinges on job performance, ability to perform adequate self-care, and overall quality of life, a reduction in the frequency or severity of the clinical manifestations of these disorders by exercise would have a substantial personal, medical, economic, and social impact.

Most of the data cited in support of the idea that an increase in physical activity increases productivity by preventing certain diseases have been derived from observational or experimental studies of the relationship between exercise and specific biologic changes linked directly or indirectly to health. These measures include indices of physical performance (e.g., endurance capacity, muscle strength, flexibility) or biologic changes not necessarily linked to improved performance (e.g., altered lipoprotein profiles, enhanced fibrinolytic activity, increased insulin sensitivity). It should not be assumed that an apparently beneficial change in any of these biological functions causes an improvement in health status, yet these relationships have substantially contributed to the impression that exercise helps prevent certain diseases.

Nearly all of the studies establishing a relationship between physical activity and clinical manifestations of disease have been observational: The health status of physically active people was compared with that of their less active counterparts (cross-sectional), or the development of disease was analyzed according to initial physical activity status (longitudinal). Very few experimental studies have been performed that have systematically investigated the influence of an increase in physical activity on the primary prevention of a specific disease other than ischemic heart disease. Available data on the relation of physical activity to the prevention of disorders such as hypertension, stroke, diabetes, or osteoporosis are mostly from observational, not experimental, studies. The nature of these studies prohibits determination of a cause-and-effect relation between physical activity and disease prevention.

The Exercise Stimulus for Disease Prevention

What biologic changes have to take place as a result of an increase in physical activity so that an improvement in health status occurs? If physical activity causes specific health benefits, then some defined stimulus must take place as a result of performing the exercise. Is the stimulus acute, occurring during and for a short time after a single bout or multiple bouts of exercise, or a longer-term "training response," occurring only after repeated bouts of exercise? The stimulus for a specific health benefit could be chemical, physical, situational, social, or a combination of these. Although much is known about the biologic changes resulting from exercise, little is known about their controlling mechanisms or the exact stimuli required to produce them.

The criterion used most frequently to evaluate the likelihood that a specific exercise training program will improve health status is whether or not it produces an increase in aerobic power. If aerobic power or another measure of endurance capacity does not significantly increase, the exercise regimen is considered unlikely to have any beneficial health effects. An increase in aerobic power is closely tied to various hemodynamic and metabolic changes produced by exercise, but many other biologic or psychologic changes may occur with exercise that do not lead to enhanced aerobic power. For example, strength training will stimulate retention of bone mineral content, increase muscle and connective tissue strength, and possibly improve psychological well-being (reduce depression, improve self-image); lower intensity endurance-type exercise ($<$ 45% $\dot{V}O_2max$) may contribute to weight control, reduce mental stress, or improve biochemical reactions important to improved health; and flexibility exercises may contribute to better musculoskeletal integrity with increasing age. It is important to maintain a very open mind when considering what exercise regimen needs to be followed to improve health.

Acute Versus Chronic Effects of Exercise

Numerous biochemical changes occur during or immediately after sustained exercise. Even though these changes may be transient, if they occur often enough they could favorably alter the progression of a specific disease or its clinical manifestations. For example, a single 45-min bout of moderate intensity endurance exercise will substantially decrease plasma triglyceride concentration if it is elevated prior to exercise (Gyntelberg, Brennan, Holloszy, Schonfeld, Rennie, & Weldman, 1977). Similar exercise on consecutive days further lowers the triglyceride concentration for 48 to 72 hr, but if exercise is not performed for several days it will return to its elevated value. This decrease in triglyceride concentration is most likely due to a rapid increase in lipoprotein lipase activity (Lithell, Orlander, & Shele, 1975), as well as to a possible reduction in hepatic triglyceride production (Zavaroni, Chen, Mondon, & Reaven, 1981). An acute response also has been reported for enhanced insulin action following 60 min of riding a cycle ergometer at 64% of $\dot{V}O_2$max (Mikines, Sonne, Farrell, Tronier, & Galbo, 1988). An increase in insulin action on glucose uptake was observed immediately and 48 hr after exercise but not 5 days after exercise. Other short-term biochemical responses to exercise that might delay the progression of disease include increased fibrinolysis or decreased platelet aggregation (Astrup, 1973).

Little is known about the intensity or duration of exercise needed to stimulate these alterations or if they directly affect the disease process, but they might represent a mechanism by which frequent exercise influences health status and productivity without necessarily producing a long-term training effect. It could be that exercise, by simply placing the body in a slightly negative caloric balance for some period of time each day, alters various metabolic functions in a way that favorably impacts the progression of disease or its clinical manifestations.

Displayed in Figure 2 are several possible patterns for acute responses to exercise that might have favorable health consequences. In panel 2-A is a response pattern in which the variable increases during exercise and returns to the preexercise value over the course of a few hours. If exercise is performed once daily or less frequently, approximately the same response would occur during and following each exercise bout. If the variable being altered in this type of response were closely linked to disease progression, exercise might provide some clinical benefit. In panel 2-B is depicted a response pattern in which the effects of one bout of exercise are carried over to the next bout when the next bout is performed the following day. In this model the magnitude of the change is influenced by the preexercise value, and the period of time the change remains is partly dependent on the magnitude of the change during exercise. Such a response pattern could readily produce significant changes in metabolic

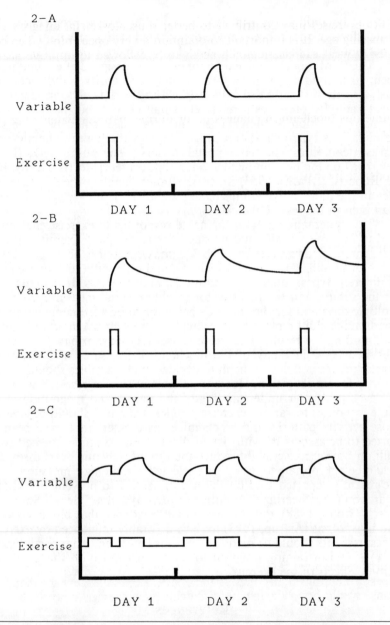

Figure 2. Examples of possible patterns of active responses to exercise of various physiologic or biochemical variables that may influence the progression of chronic degenerative disease. See text for discussion.

or hemodynamic status and significantly alter disease progression. The acute effects of endurance exercise on elevated fasting plasma triglyceride concentration appear to fit this model (Gyntelberg et al., 1977).

The third model, depicted in panel 2-C, is designed after what might occur in individuals who perform moderate intensity activity continuously or intermittently throughout much of the day. Here moderate intensity activity produces a relatively small change, but because of the extensive duration of the exercise, the total effect could be quite substantial. This type of response might explain the lower ischemic heart disease death rates reported in postal carriers versus postal clerks (Kahn, 1963) or London bus conductors versus bus drivers (Morris, Heady, Raffle, Roberts, & Parks, 1953). In these studies there is little evidence that men in the more active groups have a significantly higher aerobic power than men in the less active category.

The systematic study of the acute responses to exercise that might lead to improved health and productivity is complex. Exercise of moderate intensity or greater ($> 40\%$ $\dot{V}O_2$max) produces acute changes in numerous biologic functions which respond differently to exercise bouts of different types, intensities, durations, and intervals. It is demanding for the subject and the investigator to obtain serial measurements over multiple days and for the subject's behavior to be adequately controlled (food intake, fluid replacement, exercise, mental stress) in order to avoid confounding the results. Because a causal relationship has not been established between many of the biochemical measures of interest and disease prevention, it is difficult to decide which variables should receive priority for investigation. However, a fruitful area of research would be to develop a better understanding of the nature and magnitude of the acute responses to various exercise profiles. Attention should be given to those activity patterns and biochemical parameters that have been reported to be associated with risk of disease. For example, to shed some light on how exercise might reduce the rate of ischemic heart disease, it would be appropriate to investigate selected hematologic measures given the recently reported trial on the use of aspirin to prevent myocardial infarction (The Steering Committee of the Physicians' Health Study Research Group, 1988) and the preliminary evidence that blood viscosity and fibrinolysis (Astrup, 1973) may be favorably influenced by exercise. Measurements should be made on subjects before and after participation in an exercise training program to try to sort out both the acute and chronic effects of the exercise.

References

Astrup, T. (1973). The effects of physical activity on blood coagulation and fibrinolysis. In J.P. Naughton & H.K. Hellerstein (Eds.), *Exercise testing and exercise training and coronary heart disease* (pp. 169–192). New York: Academic Press.

Atha, J. (1981). Strengthening muscle. *Exercise and Sport Science Reviews, 9*, 1–73.

Bouchard, C. (1986). Genetics of aerobic power and capacity. In R.M. Malina & C. Bouchard (Eds.), *Sport and human genetics. The 1984 Olympic Scientific Congress Proceedings* (Vol. 4, pp. 59–88). Champaign, IL: Human Kinetics.

Bouchard, C. (1988). Gene-environment interaction in human adaptability. In *Physical activity in early and modern populations* (pp. 56–66). Champaign, IL: Human Kinetics.

DeBusk, R., Hakanssan, U., Sheehan, M., & Haskell, W. (1988). Training effects of short versus long bouts of exercise (abstract). *Journal of the American College of Cardiology, 11,* 101A.

Gaesser, G.A., & Rich, R.G. (1984). Effects of high- and low-intensity exercise training on aerobic capacity and blood lipids. *Medical Science in Sports and Exercise, 16,* 269–274.

Gossard, D., Haskell, W.L., Taylor, C.B., Muller, J.K., Rogers, F., Chandler, M., Ahn, D., Miller, N., & DeBusk, R. (1986). Effects of low- and high-intensity home-based exercise training on functional capacity in healthy middle-aged men. *American Journal of Cardiology, 57,* 446–449.

Gyntelberg, F., Brennan, R., Holloszy, J., Schonfeld, G., Rennie, M., & Weldman, S. (1977). Plasma triglyceride lowering by exercise despite increased food intake in patients with Type IV hyperlipoproteinemia. *American Journal of Clinical Nutrition, 30,* 716–720.

Kahn, H.A. (1963). The relationship of reported coronary heart disease mortality to physical activity of work. *American Journal of Public Health, 53,* 1058–1069.

Lithell, H., Orlander, J., & Shele, R. (1975). Changes in lipoprotein lipase activity and lipid stores in human skeletal muscle with prolonged heavy exercise. *Acta Physiologica Scandinavica, 107,* 257–261.

Mikines, K.J., Sonne, B., Farrell, P., Tronier, B.,& Galbo, H. (1988). Effect of physical exercise on sensitivity and responsiveness to insulin in humans. *American Journal of Physiology, 254 (Endrinol. Metab., 17),* E248–E259.

Morris, J.N., Heady, J.A., Raffle, P.A.B., Roberts, C.G., & Parks, J.W. (1953). Coronary heart disease and physical activity of work. *Lancet,* **1053,** 1111–1120.

Pollock, M. (1973). The quantification of endurance training programs. In J.W. Wilmore (Ed.), *Exercise and sport sciences reviews* (Vol. 1, pp. 155–187). New York: Academic Press.

Pollock, M.L., Miller, H.S., Janeway, R., Linnerud, A.C., Robertson, B., & Valentino, R. (1971). Effects of walking on body composition and cardiovascular function of middle-aged men. *Journal of Applied Physiology, 30,* 125–130.

Saltin, B., Blomqvist, G., Mitchell, J., Johnson, R., Wildenthal, K., & Chapman, C. (1968). Response to exercise after bed rest and after training. *Circulation, 38*(Suppl. 7), 1–78.

Skinner, J.S. (1987). *Exercise testing and exercise prescription for special cases* (pp. 101–280). Philadelphia, Lea & Febiger.

Smith, N., Ogilvie, B., Haskell, W., & Gaillard, B. (1978). *Handbook for the young athlete.* Palo Alto, CA: Bull Publishing.

The Steering Committee of the Physicians' Health Study Research Group. (1988). Preliminary report: Findings from the Aspirin Component of the ongoing Physicians' Health Study. *New England Journal of Medicine, 4,* 262–264.

Wood, P.W., Terry, R., & Haskell, W. (1985). Metabolism of substrates: Diet, lipoprotein metabolism and exercise. *Federation Proceedings, 44,* 358–363.

Zavaroni, I., Chen, Y-D., Mondon, C.E., & Reaven, G.M. (1981). Ability of exercise to inhibit carbohydrate induced hypertriglyceridemia in rats. *Metabolism, 30,* 476–480.

The Psychological Effects of Exercise

Judith Rodin and Thomas Plante
Yale University
New Haven, Connecticut

Thousands of businesses in the United States have implemented programs to promote physical fitness among their employees (Falkenberg, 1987). The programs range from company-paid memberships at private health and fitness clubs to complete work site fitness facilities. These programs have been developed not only to improve and maintain employee health but also to promote psychological well-being and productivity and to reduce absenteeism, insurance claims, and stress. Recent research focusing on the use of employee fitness programs to improve work-related behaviors suggests that these programs may improve absenteeism, job satisfaction, tenure, and health care costs, especially among female employees (Baun, Bernacki, & Tsai, 1986; Bernacki & Baun, 1984; Browne, Russell, Morgan, Optenberg, & Clarke, 1984; Der-Karabetian & Gebharp, 1986; Tsai, Baun, & Bernacki, 1987).

If cost-effective outcomes result from the implementation of corporate fitness programs, it becomes important to identify the psychological and physiological changes that produce these effects. This paper reviews recent data considering possible psychological benefits of exercise.

Numerous articles have been published in the professional and popular presses extolling the virtues of regular physical exercise. The exercise boom of the 1970s saw a substantial increase in the number of people engaged in aerobic exercise, such as running and aerobic dancing (Cooper, 1982). The popular notion is that exercise enhances mood, self-concept, and general psychological well-being. People commonly report a reliance on exercise as a means of maintaining a wealth of psychological benefits.

Given these various claims, it is surprising that only a small proportion of scientific studies have examined the psychological effects of exercise among normal, nonclinically disturbed populations. Instead, the professional literature has focused on exercise as a clinical intervention. This review highlights those research studies that considered the psychological consequences of exercise in nonclinical populations since the publication of a past review article (Folkins & Sime, 1981). We excluded

127

studies that were severely methodologically flawed, for example, that failed to use control groups or used anecdotal case studies. Four areas of psychological functioning have been most widely examined in recent research. These include (a) psychological well-being and mood, (b) mild anxiety and stress, (c) personality and self-concept, and (d) cognition.

Psychological Well-Being and Mood

In seeking to understand the beneficial effects of exercise and how they are produced, it is important to consider separately what happens to mood and well-being immediately after an exercise workout and what the longer-term benefits are of maintaining an exercise regimen. Two studies support the notion that physical activity improves mood and well-being immediately following an exercise workout. Lichtman and Posner (1983) studied 32 exercise class subjects at a local YMCA and 32 community college hobby class subjects matched for age. Although both exercise and hobby activities were associated with mood improvement, physical activity had a stronger association. Berger and Owen (1983) examined 36 beginning and intermediate college swim class members and 42 students attending physical education and health sciences lecture classes as controls. Results demonstrated that the swimmers experienced significantly improved mood relative to the control group immediately following their class.

Goldwater and Collis (1985) considered longer-term improvements in mood and well-being following participation in an exercise program. They selected 51 nonexercising volunteers from a university setting and randomly assigned them to an aerobic exercise group ($n = 27$) or a pseudo-exercise control group ($n = 24$) designed to "minimize . . . cardiovascular (conditioning) . . . while still giving the appearance of a conditioning program" (p. 177). Results demonstrated significant improvements in anxiety and well-being for the exercise group relative to the control group. A number of other studies have also supported the connection between exercise and well-being and/or mood (Brown & Lawton, 1986; Ewing & Scott, 1984; Hayes & Ross, 1986). Due to methodological considerations, however, the results and conclusions of these studies must be viewed with caution.

In summary, empirical research conducted since 1980 suggests that exercise improves mood and well-being immediately following an exercise workout. Although there is some evidence for improvement in general mood and well-being as a result of participating in a long-term exercise program, support for these long-term, cumulative effects is not as compelling as the evidence for the immediate effects of exercise on improved mood and well-being.

Mild Anxiety, Depression, and Stress

Five studies that concentrated specifically on reductions in anxiety, depression, and/or stress among nonclinical subjects met our methodological criteria. Two used experimental manipulations by having some subjects participate in exercise programs over several weeks while the remaining subjects were assigned to control conditions (Blumenthal, Williams, Needels, & Wallace, 1982; Lobitz, Brammel, Stoll & Niccoli, 1983). Three used correlational methods to test the hypothesis that anxiety (Hayden & Allen, 1984; Sothmann & Ismail, 1984) and depression (Hayden & Allen, 1984; Lobstein, Mosbacher, & Ismail, 1983; Sothmann & Ismail, 1984) were lower in physically active adults than in sedentary ones. Four of these studies found significant reductions in stress, anxiety, and/or depression among exercisers (Blumenthal et al., 1982; Hayden & Allen, 1984; Lobitz et al., 1983; Lobstein et al., 1984).

Eight additional studies have explored the relationship between physical fitness and mild anxiety, depression, and stress (Farrell, Gustafson, Morgan, & Pert, 1987; Parent & Whall, 1984; Pauly, Palmer, Wright, & Pfeiffer, 1982; Perri & Templer, 1985; Severtsen & Bruya, 1986; Tucker, Cole, & Freidman, 1986; Valliant & Asu, 1985; Wilfley & Kunce, 1986). Although these studies have methodological flaws that preclude confidence in their results and conclusions, seven of them concluded that exercise is associated with less anxiety, depression, and/or stress. The data thus support the belief that exercise is effective in reducing negative emotional states. Here both the immediate and longer-term benefits of exercise seem apparent.

Personality and Self-Concept

With so much attention given to findings that the hard-driving, competitive, Type A personality may be at greater risk for coronary heart disease (Friedman et al., 1986; Rosenman et al., 1975), recent studies have attempted to change aspects of this behavior pattern. Two have used aerobic exercise programs as the intervention and compared the exercise to the effects of stress management training (Lobitz et al., 1983; Roskies et al., 1986). Both studies found benefits for both the aerobic training and stress management interventions, but only Lobitz et al. found reductions in Type A behavior. Recent studies have suggested that only the potential for the hostility component (Dembroski & Costa, 1987) and the anger component (Booth-Kewley & Friedman, 1987) of the Type A personality are risk factors for coronary heart disease. Certain types of exercise (e.g., rapid, intense, energetic workouts on training machines) may work better than others to release pent-up anger and hostility. Lobitz et al. used this type of training, whereas Roskies et al. used jogging.

Other potential personality and self-concept changes following exercise have also been explored. Jasnoski and Holmes (1981) studied 103 college females before and after a 15-week aerobic training program. After statistically controlling for the effects of changes in aerobic conditioning they found that participation in the program resulted in subjects appearing less inhibited, more imaginative, and more self-assured. Greater aerobic performance was also significantly associated with more free-thinking and less tension. These data suggest that although improved physical fitness itself is associated with changes, factors related to being involved in fitness training per se are also related to improved self-concept. Other studies also support the conclusion that being involved with and committed to an exercise program improves self-concept and self-esteem (Parent & Whall, 1984; Pauly et al., 1982; Perri & Templer, 1985; Valliant & Asu, 1985).

Cognitive Processes

Studies comparing the test performance of subjects differing in physical fitness during and after exercise of short duration and moderate intensity (e.g., Sjoberg, 1980) support the view that cognitive function is facilitated by an increase in physical arousal. Also, physically fit individuals are better able to perform cognitive tasks while under moderate levels of physical stress than are less physically fit individuals. The effects of long-duration aerobic exercise are less clear, however. Tomporowski, Ellis, and Stephens (1985) studied subjects of low, moderate, and high fitness after each group had engaged in a strenuous run. No differential effects for any group, compared with a no-exercise control group, were found for performance on a memory task.

In summary, it appears that exercise may initially facilitate attentional processes; however, as exercise intensity and duration increase, the facilitative effects of exercise may be canceled by the debilitating effects of muscular fatigue. A full review of this literature has recently been published (Tomporowski & Ellis, 1986).

Implications for Work Performance

If exercise improves performance, psychological well-being, mood, and self-concept and reduces mild anxiety and stress, as the research reviewed suggests, exercisers may prove to be better employees than nonexercisers. One could predict that if exercising employees are more psychologically and physically healthy relative to nonexercising employees, they would be more likely to be productive and satisfied with their jobs, be less likely to have high absenteeism or health care costs, and appear generally more well-adjusted in the workplace. But what actually changes psychologically as a function of exercise that is important for the work environment?

The short-term benefits of just having engaged in aerobic exercise seem most clearly due to the effects of aerobic activity per se. Fitness centers in the workplace make sense if employees return to work with elevated mood, less tension, and improved cognitive activity. It appears that performance in the workplace can be improved by the psychological gains derived from an aerobic exercise workout, in particular.

The long-term benefits of aerobic exercise per se for psychological well-being and performance seem less clear. Until now many investigators have considered aerobic training, resulting in a measurable increase in oxygen uptake, to be necessary for longer-term psychological changes. However, results of two well-controlled prospective trials fail to support the hypothesis that changes in aerobic fitness levels are associated with changes in psychological health items (Hughes, 1984; King, Taylor, Haskell, & DeBusk, in press). In addition, at least one recent experimentally controlled study of the effects of systematic exercise training on clinical depression found significant reductions in depression relative to waiting list controls for participants engaging in both aerobic (running) and non-aerobic (weight lifting) activities (Doyne et al., 1987). Such findings call into question the mechanisms through which exercise may exert its influence on psychological state in the long run.

Until recently, investigators have not considered the possibility that many positive results may accrue because of psychological gains experienced from trying to get fit rather than, or at least in addition to, gains attributable to physical fitness per se. Yet the rapidity of the changes reported in most studies suggests that factors other than those stemming from improved physical conditioning are likely to be responsible. For example, perceived fitness, which is often uncorrelated with actual changes in $\dot{V}O_2$max (King et al., in press) may be the crucial variable leading to improved psychological changes. A similar finding in another domain showed that perceived health was a better predictor of mortality 20 years later than any of the "harder" physiological variables, including measurable cardiovascular health (Kaplan & Camacho, 1983). To a degree, the psychological meaning of engaging in exercise may be as important as the physical benefits.

Why might these perceived variables be the crucial mediators between engaging in exercise and positive psychological effects? Among the types of thoughts that affect human motivation and action, none is more central or pervasive than those concerning personal efficacy. Perceived self-efficacy refers to beliefs in one's capabilities to execute the competencies needed to have control over events that affect one's welfare. My work (Rodin, 1986) and Bandura's (1986) have shown that self-efficacy plays a central role in human behavior. People's feelings of control affect their sense of choice regarding the courses of action they wish to pursue. When people feel efficacious, they are likely to mobilize considerably more effort, that is, to appear more motivated and to persevere in the face of obstacles and failure experiences. People who regard themselves as highly efficacious set themselves challenges and intensify their efforts when their performances fall short of their goals. Perceived control leads to a sense of task importance and commitment. Such self-assured endeavor produces accomplishments.

It is possible that viewing oneself as physically fit or having the self-image of an exerciser influences self-efficacy because exercise requires effort and commitment. Getting fit is hard work. Of course, good physical conditioning itself may enhance one's sense of efficacy, but it is possible that there is an additional gain. Engaging in exercise itself may lead to an increased sense of power and self-determination.

In order to assess these hypotheses, we selected individuals who were not aerobically fit and had not engaged in any systematic exercise program for at least 2 years and assigned them at random to one of four experimental conditions (Rodin, unpublished data). In two groups, subjects went through two exercise classes per week for 12 weeks. The other two groups had language classes of the same duration for the same number of weeks. One exercise group and one language group were given repeated information over the course of the several weeks of training that what they were doing was extremely difficult and that few people were able to achieve what they had achieved in so short a time. Other such encouragement continued throughout the sessions. This encouragement was intended to give subjects an increased sense of self-efficacy: that what they were doing was something difficult, something that they should feel proud about, and something that few others could do quite as well. No direct manipulations of efficacy were provided for the other two groups.

Measures of self-efficacy showed that the manipulations were highly successful (see Figure 1). Subjects in the high-efficacy conditions had significantly and uniformly higher levels of perceived self-efficacy from before to after the training. The results on all categories of psychological variables described earlier showed significant improvement for the high-efficacy groups. As Figure 2 demonstrates, there were substantial improvements in mood and psychological well-being, reductions in anxiety and stress, increased self-concept, and increased performance on cognitive tasks. Within the high-efficacy conditions, the effects of high experienced efficacy were greater for the exercise than for the language group on some variables.

These data suggest that high perceived control does produce the gains in psychological well-being and performance that have been studied in the exercise literature, regardless of the type of task that induces the sense of efficacy. Thus, when exercise enhances self-efficacy, its benefits may

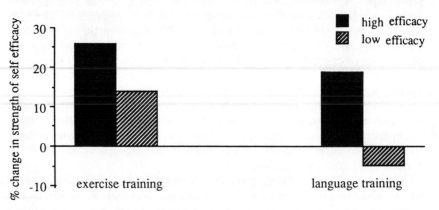

Figure 1.   Percent change in perceptions of self-efficacy from before to after exercise and language training. High and low efficacy groups refer to manipulations intended to influence perceived efficacy.

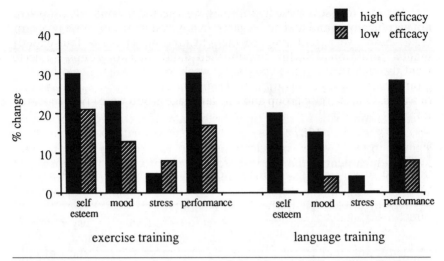

Figure 2. Percent change in measures of the effects of differential self-efficacy among subjects in the exercise training and language training groups. Measures include self-esteem, mood, stress, and performance on a memory task.

be above and beyond effects due to improvement in fitness per se. Over time, however, the two most likely become mutually reinforcing domains. As individuals feel more efficacious and better about themselves, they are willing to exercise more and to persist in exercise regimens. This can improve their overall fitness because persistence and motivation to exercise are crucial to long-term gains in conditioning. Our weight control studies suggest that even people who only do jumping jacks for 10 minutes a day three times a week are substantially more successful at weight control. Clearly we cannot attribute these effects to increased metabolic rate or increased physical expenditure alone when the type and amount of exercise is so minimal. Quite likely these people, seeing themselves as "exercisers" who were doing something about their health, actually restricted their food intake more, particularly of high-calorie foods. Thus the psychological meaning of exercise is central.

There are many other psychological benefits of exercise that have not yet been fully explored. For example, exercise may improve one's sense of optimism. Optimism, as defined by Webster's dictionary, is an inclination to anticipate the best possible outcome. Since the influence of Norman Cousins and before him Norman Vincent Peale, there has been popular interest in the power of positive thinking. But only recently has scientific attention been devoted to the possibility that optimism may confer beneficial effects. This work, like studies investigating the effects of perceived control, is based on the assumption that people's actions are greatly affected by their beliefs about the probable outcomes of these actions.

Recent evidence has suggested that a person's sense of optimism seems to promote a higher level of physical well-being. For example, studies by Recker and Wong (1985) and Scheier and Carver (1985) found that optimists report fewer physical symptoms and more positive physical, psychological, and general well-being. Indeed, Scheier and Carver and their coworkers recently showed that optimists, as determined prior to coronary artery bypass surgery, were judged by members of the cardiac rehabilitation team as showing a faster rate of recovery (described in Scheier & Carver, 1987). They used fewer pain medications, had fewer signs of intraoperative complications, and showed much better psychological adjustment to the surgical procedures. Pilot work that we are just completing suggests that exercise increases one's sense of optimism. If so, there is another mechanism whereby the psychological gains from exercise may have tangible physical health benefits.

Many other theories have also been offered to explain psychological improvements resulting from exercise. One states that exercise is a form of meditation that triggers an altered and more relaxed state of consciousness (e.g., Buffone, 1980). Another proposes that exercise is a form of biofeedback that teaches exercisers to regulate their own autonomic arousal (e.g., Hollandsworth, 1979). Another theory suggests that exercise provides distraction, diversion, or time-out from unpleasant cognitions, emotions, and behaviors (e.g., Long, 1983). It has also been suggested that exercise has beneficial effects because it produces the physical symptoms associated with anxiety and stress (e.g., sweating, hyperventilation, fatigue) without the subjective experience of emotional distress. Repeated pairing of the symptoms in the absence of associated distress results in improved psychological functioning (Hughes, 1984). Finally, the substantial social reinforcement afforded exercisers may also lead to improved psychological states (Hughes). Although I favor the power and optimism explanations, at present no single theory or group of theories has been confirmed with sufficient scientific evidence. Systematic studies are needed to test these alternative perspectives.

References

Bandura, A. (1986). From thought to action: Mechanisms of personal agency. *New Zealand Journal of Psychology, 15,* 1–17.

Baun, W.B., Bernacki, E.J., & Tsai, S.P. (1986). A preliminary investigation: Effect of a corporate fitness program on absenteeism and health care cost. *Journal of Occupational Medicine, 28,* 18–20.

Berger, B.G., & Owen, D.R. (1983). Mood alteration with swimming: Swimmers really do "feel better." *Psychosomatic Medicine, 45,* 425–433.

Bernacki, E.J., & Baun, W.B. (1984). The relationship of job performance to exercise adherence in a corporate fitness program. *Journal of Occupational Medicine, 26,* 529–531.

Blumenthal, J.A., Williams, S., Needels, T.L., & Wallace, A.G. (1982). Psychological changes accompany aerobic exercise in healthy middle-aged adults. *Psychosomatic Medicine, 44,* 529–535.

Booth-Kewley, S., & Friedman, H.S. (1987). Psychological predictors of heart disease: A quantitative review. *Psychology Bulletin, 101,* 343–362.

Brown, J.D., & Lawton, M. (1986). Stress and well-being in adolescence: The moderating role of physical exercise. *Journal of Human Stress, 12,* 125–131.

Browne, D.W., Russell, M.L., Morgan, J.L., Optenberg, S.A., & Clarke, A.E. (1984). Reduced disability and health care costs in an industrial fitness program. *Journal of Occupational Medicine, 26,* 809–816.

Buffone, G.W. (1980). Exercise as therapy: A closer look. *Journal of Counseling and Psychotherapy, 3,* 101–105.

Cooper, K.H. (1982). The aerobic program for total well being. New York: Bantam.

Dembroski, T.M., & Costa, P.T., Jr. (1987). Coronary prone behavior: Components of the type A pattern and hostility. *Journal of Personality, 55,* 211–235.

Der-Karabetian, A., & Gebharp, N. (1986). Effect of physical fitness program in the workplace. *Journal of Business and Psychology, 1,* 51–57.

Doyne, E.J., Ossip-Klein, D.J., Bowman, E.D., Osborn, K.M., McDougall-Wilson, I.B., & Neimeyer, R.A. (1987). Running versus weight lifting in the treatment of depression. *Journal of Consulting and Clinical Psychology, 55,* 748–754.

Ewing, J.H., & Scott, D.G. (1984). Effects of aerobic exercise upon affect and cognition. *Perceptual and Motor Skills, 59,* 407–414.

Falkenberg, L.E. (1987). Employee fitness programs: Their impact on the employee and the organization. *Academy of Management Review, 12,* 511–521.

Farrell, P.A., Gustafson, A.B., Morgan, W.P., & Pert, C.B. (1987). Enkephalins, catecholamines, and psychological mood alterations: Effects of prolonged exercise. *Medicine and Science in Sports and Exercise, 19,* 347–353.

Folkins, C.H., & Sime, W.E. (1981). Physical fitness and mental health. *American Psychologist, 36,* 373–389.

Friedman, M., Thoresen, C.E., Gill, J.J., Ulmer, D., Powell, L.H., Price, V.A., Brown, B., Thompson, L., Rabin, D.D., Breall, W.S., Bourg, E., Levy, R., & Dixon, T. (1986). Alteration of type A behavior and its effect on cardiac recurrences in post myocardial infarction patients: Summary results of the recurrent coronary prevention project. *American Heart Journal, 112,* 653–665.

Goldwater, B.C., & Collis, M.L. (1985). Psychologic effects of cardiovascular conditioning: A controlled experiment. *Psychosomatic Medicine, 47,* 174–181.

Hayden, R.M., & Allen, G.J. (1984). Relationship between aerobic exercise, anxiety, and depression: Convergent validation by knowledgeable informants. *Journal of Sports Medicine, 24,* 69–74.

Hayes, D., & Ross, C.E. (1986). Body and mind: The effect of exercise, overweight, and physical health and psychological well-being. *Journal of Health and Social Behavior,* **27,** 387–400.

Hollandsworth, J.G. (1979). Some thoughts on distance running as training in biofeedback. *Journal of Sport Behavior,* **2,** 71–82.

Hughes, J.R. (1984). Psychological effects of habitual aerobic exercise: A critical review. *Preventive Medicine,* **13,** 66–78.

Jasnoski, M.L., & Holmes, D.S. (1981). Influence of initial aerobic fitness, aerobic training and changes in aerobic fitness on personality functioning. *Journal of Psychosomatic Research,* **25,** 553–556.

Kaplan, G.A., & Camacho, T. (1983). Perceived health and mortality: A nine-year follow-up of the human population laboratory cohort. *American Journal of Epidemiology,* **117,** 292–304.

King, A.C., Taylor, C.B., Haskell, W.L., & DeBusk, R.F. (in press). The influence of regular aerobic exercise on psychological health: A randomized, controlled trial of healthy middle-aged adults. *Health Psychology.*

Lichtman, S., & Posner, E.G. (1983). The effects of exercise on mood and cognitive functioning. *Journal of Psychosomatic Research,* **27,** 43–52.

Lobitz, W.C., Brammel, H.L., Stoll, S., & Niccoli, A. (1983). Physical exercise and anxiety management training for cardiac stress management in a nonpatient population. *Journal of Cardiac Rehabilitation,* **3,** 683–688.

Lobstein, D.D., Mosbacher, B.J., & Ismail, A.H. (1983). Depression as a powerful discriminator between physically active and sedentary middle-aged men. *Journal of Psychosomatic Research,* **27,** 69–76.

Long, B.C. (1983). Aerobic conditioning and stress reduction: Participation or conditioning? *Human Movement Science,* **2,** 171–186.

Parent, C.J., & Whall, A.L. (1984). Are physical activity, self-esteem, and depression related? *Journal of Gerontological Nursing,* **10,** 8–10.

Pauly, J.T., Palmer, J.A., Wright, C.C., & Pfeiffer, G.J. (1982). The effect of a 14-week employee fitness program on selected physiological and psychological parameters. *Journal of Occupational Medicine,* **24,** 457–463.

Perri, S., & Templer, D.I. (1985). The effects of an aerobic exercise program on psychological variables in older adults. *International Journal of Aging and Human Development,* **20,** 167–172.

Recker, G.T., & Wong, P.T.P. (1985). Personal optimism, physical and mental health: The triumph of successful aging. In J.E. Birren and J. Livingston (Eds.)., *Cognition, stress and aging.* New York: Prentice-Hall.

Rodin, J. (1986). Aging and health. Effects of the sense of control. *Science,* **233,** 1271–1276.

Rosenman, R.H., Brand, R.J., Jenkins, C.D., Friedman, M., Straus, R., & Wurm, M. (1975). Coronary heart disease in the Western Collaborative Group study: Final follow-up experience of 8 1/2 years. *Journal of the American Medical Association,* **233,** 872–877.

Roskies, E., Seraganian, P., Oseasohn, R., Hanley, J.A., Collu, R., Martin, N., & Smilga, C. (1986). The Montreal Type A intervention project: Major findings. *Health Psychology, 5*, 45–69.

Scheier, M.F., & Carver, C.S. (1985). Optimism, coping, and health: Assessment and implications of generalized outcome expectancies. *Health Psychology, 4*, 219–247.

Scheier, M.F., & Carver, C.S. (1987). Dispositional optimism and physical well-being: The influence of generalized outcome expectancies on health. *Journal of Personality, 55*, 169–210.

Severtsen, B., & Bruya, M.A. (1986). Effects of meditation and aerobic exercise on EEG patterns. *Journal of Neuroscience Nursing, 18*, 206–210.

Sjoberg, H. (1980). Physical fitness and mental performance during and after work. *Ergonomics, 23*, 977–995.

Sothmann, M.S., & Ismail, A.H., (1984). Relationship between urinary catecholamine metabolites, particularly MHPG, and selected personality and physical fitness characteristics in normal subjects. *Psychosomatic Medicine, 46*, 523–531.

Tomporowski, P.D., Ellis, N.R., & Stephens, R. (1985). *The immediate effects of aerobic exercise on free-recall memory.* In P.D. Tomporowski & N.R. Ellis, *Psychological Bulletin, 99*, 338–348.

Tomporowski, P.D., & Ellis, N.R. (1986). Effects of exercise on cognitive processes: A review. *Psychological Bulletin, 99*, 338–346.

Tsai, S.P., Baun, W.B., & Bernacki, E.J. (1987). Relationship of employee turnover to exercise adherence in a corporate fitness program. *Journal of Occupational Medicine, 29*, 572–575.

Tucker, L.A., Cole, G.E., & Friedman, G.M. (1986). Physical fitness: A buffer against stress. *Perceptual and Motor Skills, 61*, 1031–1038.

Valliant, P.M., & Asu, M.E. (1985). Exercise and its effects on cognition and physiology in older adults. *Perceptual and Motor Skills, 63*, 955–961.

Wilfley, D., & Kunce, J. (1986). Differential physical and psychological effects of exercise. *Journal of Counseling Psychology, 63*(3), 337–342.

Frontiers of Exercise Research: A Search for the Molecular Basis of the Exercise Training Effect in Skeletal Muscle

R. Sanders Williams
Duke University Medical Center
Durham, North Carolina

The participants in this conference raised many provocative and important questions concerning the relationships between physical activity and biological fitness. The discussions demonstrated that valuable new directions of exercise research lie in many dimensions: behavioral and sociological as well as physiological and biochemical. However, in my opinion, one of the most exciting frontiers of exercise research is based on the concept that many of the physiologically important adaptive responses to physical activity can be considered as questions of gene regulation.

Physical activity leads to greater expression of certain genes and diminished expression of other genes within several types of cells. When fundamental questions that are important to a greater understanding of the biological effects of physical activity are posed as problems of gene regulation, they may be answerable by application of powerful new experimental techniques that have arisen from recent advances in molecular genetics. In my laboratory, we have chosen this approach to a central question of exercise research: What are the molecular signaling pathways by which changes in tonic contractile activity result in increased expression of proteins of oxidative metabolism in skeletal muscles? The discussion that follows will illustrate a theoretical framework that we are using to select specific experiments that may bring us closer to an answer to this question. Our emphasis on the cell and the molecular biology of exercise is based upon two premises: first, that greater understanding of basic mechanisms of important physiological phenomena is in itself an important goal, and, second, that in the long run, fundamental knowledge of the mechanisms by which physical activity results in objective changes in cell and organ physiology will improve our ability to make rational decisions concerning the expenditure of time and money for exercise— as individuals, as corporations, and as a society.

139

Members of ancient societies were aware that habitual physical activity results in a greater capacity to perform physical work without fatigue, but only in this century have we begun to understand the biological basis of this phenomenon. Beginning with the observations that fitter individuals can consume more oxygen per unit of time and that maximal oxygen consumption can be increased by training, the changes in organ physiology, in cell physiology, in the function of subcellular organelles, and in specific biochemical pathways that permit individuals to exercise for longer durations and at greater intensities after a period of training have been defined in some detail (Holloszy & Coyle, 1984; Saltin & Gollnick, 1983). These changes involve several types of cells and tissues, but the most profound and reproducible effects are produced within the skeletal muscles that participate in the training activity.

A change in the habitual pattern of tonic contractile activity of skeletal muscles of humans or laboratory animals produces adaptations that make the muscle resistant to fatigue during sustained, repeated contractions. At a morphological level, two features of trained muscles are most evident: a greater density of capillaries relative to muscle fibers and a greater density of mitochondria within the muscle fibers (Hoppeler et al., 1985). At a biochemical level, endurance-trained muscles contain greater concentrations of proteins involved in generation of ATP via combustion of molecular oxygen (Saltin & Gollnick, 1983). These adaptations permit the muscle to meet the energy demands of sustained contractile work through oxidative rather than anaerobic metabolism, thereby reducing the rate of accumulation of lactate and permitting the muscle to employ the vast energy reserves stored in body fat rather than the limited reserves found in muscle and liver glycogen (Holloszy & Coyle, 1984).

One of the major accomplishments of exercise research up to this time is the knowledge that exercise-induced increases in the cellular content of proteins of oxidative metabolism within skeletal muscles produce many of the physiological characteristics of the trained state. It is fitting, therefore, to use this fact as a point of departure for future investigations. Most importantly, the biochemical signaling pathways by which muscle cells can sense an increase in demand for contractile activity and respond with physiologically advantageous adaptations in the cellular content of certain proteins remain almost entirely unknown. Elucidation of these pathways, therefore, is a critical frontier of exercise research.

Statement of the General Hypothesis

The general hypothesis under consideration is that repetitive contractions of a skeletal muscle result in generation of a molecular signal (X) and that the accumulation of this signal molecule results in increased synthesis of specific proteins of oxidative metabolism. The hypothesis is stated in this simple form, but it is important to recognize that more than one signal molecule may be involved and that any one signal molecule may act through pathways that involve many steps, each of which is subject to alternative pathways of regulation. If this general hypothesis is correct, what characteristics of signal X are compatible with existing knowledge about the effects of exercise training on the synthesis of proteins of oxidative metabolism in skeletal muscle?

1. *Signal X acts locally.* The effects of endurance exercise on oxidative capacity of skeletal muscles are limited, almost exclusively, to muscles that participate in the training activity (Holloszy & Coyle, 1984; Salmons & Henriksson, 1981; Saltin & Gollnick, 1983). It is clear, therefore, that signal X is not carried in the blood in a form that can exert remote effects on resting muscles and is not related directly to the changes in circulating hormones that occur during exercise with large muscle groups (Galbo, 1983). In addition, the effects of signal X appear to be relatively independent of experimentally induced variations in plasma concentrations of pituitary hormones, glucocorticoids, or thyroid hormones (Galbo; Holloszy & Coyle; Saltin & Gollnick). The relationship of signal X to the activity of catecholamines in skeletal muscles is more controversial. Administration of β-adrenergic antagonists may reduce the effects of endurance training on the content of oxidative enzymes in trained muscles, but does not abolish the responses to training (Ji, Lennon, Kochan, Nagle, & Lardy, 1986; Wolfel et al., 1986). Furthermore, repeated administration of β-adrenergic agonists has been reported to produce effects in resting skeletal muscles that are similar to the adaptations induced by endurance training (Liang, Tuttle, Hood, & Haralambos, 1979; Sullivan et al., 1985). Therefore, although circulating or neurally released catecholamines are not identical to signal X, it appears that intracellular events mediated through β-adrenergic receptors may intersect with pathways triggered by signal X.

It is unlikely that signal X is a trophic factor released from motor neurons, because direct stimulation of denervated muscles produces effects similar to those produced by nerve stimulation or endurance training (Henriksson, Galbo, & Blomstrand, 1982). It is conceivable that signal X is an autocrine or paracrine factor that is produced in one cell (probably within muscle fibers but conceivably within endothelial cells or other nonmyocyte cells within the muscle), but is released into the extracellular environment to exert its effects either upon its cell of origin or upon surrounding cells. However, it seems most plausible that signal X is produced intracellularly during contractions of skeletal muscle fibers and acts exclusively within the fiber in which it was generated.

2. *Signal X itself, or the activated state of some factor in a pathway triggered by signal X, has a long half-life, persisting for days following a brief period of contractile activity.* A remarkable feature of the response of skeletal muscle to endurance training is the manner in which a few minutes of physical activity, separated by long periods of inactivity, can produce profound effects. Within several weeks, an hour or less of submaximal exercise three to five times weekly is sufficient to induce biochemically measurable and physiologically significant increases in muscle oxidative capacity (Holloszy & Coyle, 1984; Saltin & Gollnick, 1983). Thus, even through a single brief period of exercise has no measurable

effect, it alters the muscle fibers in some way so that further periods of exercise produce an incremental and cumulative response.

3. Signal X itself, or the activated state of some factor in a pathway triggered by signal X, accumulates slowly, even when the stimulus to generation of signal X is maximal. Studies of human volunteers or animals indicate that several weeks are required before training-induced increments in muscle content of oxidative enzymes can be detected (Holloszy & Coyle, 1984; Saltin & Gollnick 1983). Even in experimental animals in which continuous contractile activity is produced by continuous motor nerve stimulation for 12 to 24 hr daily (a protocol that may be considered a maximal stimulus to the generation of signal X), a latency period of several days is required before increased concentrations of oxidative enzymes are observed (Henriksson et al., 1986; Pette & Vrbova, 1985). Furthermore, this latency or lag period also is evident when levels of mRNA encoding proteins of oxidative metabolism are measured (Seedorf, Leberer, Kirschbaum, & Pette, 1986; Underwood & Williams, 1987; Williams, Garcia-Moll, Mellor, Salmons, & Harlan, 1987; Williams, Salmons, Newsholme, Kaufman, & Mellor, 1986), indicating that the delay is not simply a function of the time required for accumulation of newly synthesized proteins of oxidative metabolism after an immediate increase in the rate of protein synthesis. Thus, the response to signal X is not a simple function of the time and intensity of the stimulus. In addition, the seemingly obligatory lag period of several days that occurs between the onset of the stimulus to the generation of signal X (muscle contraction) and the response to signal X (increase in oxidative enzymes) contrasts distinctly with the time course of many other stimulus-response pathways that act upon mammalian cells (e.g., effects mediated in response to hormones or growth factors), in which responses follow stimuli by only seconds, minutes, or hours.

4. The effects of signal X are limited to proteins of oxidative metabolism and do not affect global rates of protein synthesis. By definition, the pathways that we are seeking to identify are highly selective. Changes in contractile activity are known to induce generalized effects on global rates of RNA and protein synthesis in muscle cells (Booth & Watson, 1985; Pette, 1984). Although generalized adaptive responses of this type probably have major importance as mechanisms of muscle hypertrophy in response to changes in contractile demand, our focus is upon the pathways that lead to selective effects upon the specific set of genes that encode proteins of oxidative metabolism. The cellular content of these proteins is increased by endurance training or continuous nerve stimulation in the absence of muscle hypertrophy and in the absence of increases in the cellular content of most contractile proteins, indicating that the pathways triggered by signal X do not act upon other genes in a nonspecific manner.

5. The effects of signal X act to regulate transcription of genes that encode proteins of oxidative metabolism. Pathways that regulate the cellular content of individual proteins can exert their effects at any of the multiple biochemical steps that transpire between synthesis of the primary gene transcript and assembly of functional enzymatic complexes.

The cellular content of an individual protein also can be regulated by selective changes in rates of protein degradation, but this latter mechanism does not appear to be important in the effects of tonic contractile activity upon the content of proteins of oxidative metabolism in skeletal muscles (Booth & Watson, 1985). Several laboratories have demonstrated that tonic contractile activity regulates steady-state concentrations of mRNAs encoding specific proteins of oxidative metabolism (Pluskal & Streter, 1983; Seedorf et al., 1986; Underwood & Williams, 1987; Williams et al., 1987; Williams et al., 1986). This finding can reflect either increased rates of transcription of these genes or increased stability of these specific mRNAs. However, in developing a theoretical framework for the search for signal X, I have chosen to interpret the steady-state RNA data as indicative of differences in transcriptional efficiency, recognizing that this framework may be abandoned if further experiments point to changes in message stability as the major basis for activity-induced increases in mRNA concentrations.

In developing a strategy for the search for signal X, I have chosen also to interpret the steady-state RNA data as indicating a greater role for transcriptional rather than specific translational control of expression of these genes. The assumption is reasonable for the purpose of focusing an experimental plan, but it is important to acknowledge that control at the level of translation may contribute to activity-induced changes in expression of proteins of oxidative metabolism. In model systems in which motor nerve stimulation is employed to increase the oxidative capacity of muscle fibers, changes in the specific activity of certain mitochondrial enzymes do not correspond precisely to changes in the levels of mRNA encoding mitochondrial proteins (Seedorf et al., 1986; Williams et al., 1987). At this time it is unclear whether these results merely reflect the limited precision of quantitative measurements of mRNA concentrations or truly reflect an important role for translational control mechanisms in this adaptation.

Development of Specific Hypotheses Concerning Signal X

Specific hypotheses concerning the identity of signal X should be compatible with the five characteristics described in the preceding discussion. In addition, the plausibility of any specific hypothesis would be enhanced by evidence of a similar pathway of gene regulation in response to other types of stimuli in other types of eukaryotic cells. In this regard it may be instructive to draw analogies from regulatory pathways by which lower organisms, such as yeasts, respond to changing environmental conditions by coordinated changes in expression of sets of genes that encode functionally related proteins. The molecular biology that underlies the phenomena of glucose repression, of general control of enzymes of amino acid synthesis by amino acid starvation, and of regulation of cytochrome genes by heme has been elucidated in elegant detail in S. cerevesiae (Arndt & Fink, 1986; Celenza & Carlson, 1986; Guarente & Mason, 1983; Johnston, Zavortink, Debouck, & Hopper, 1986; Xitomer et al., 1987). These studies provide models for development of hypotheses concerning the mechanisms that may function to permit mammalian muscle cells to respond to the changing environmental conditions associated with physical activity. On this basis, several more specific hypotheses to account for the effects of signal X can be formulated.

Hypothesis: The pathway triggered by signal X involves a nuclear protein factor, the activity of which regulates the transcription of a set of genes that encode proteins of oxidative metabolism.

Hypothesis: Signal X, mobilized by a period of tonic contractile activity, results in activation of this nuclear protein factor, either by increasing the rate at which it is synthesized, by inducing its translocation into the nucleus from an extranuclear compartment, by causing a stable posttranslational modification (e.g. phosphorylation or proteolytic cleavage), or by increasing the availability of a cofactor essential for its activity, the concentration of which is limited in resting muscle.

If these hypotheses are correct, the concentrations of signal X itself may be increased only transiently during a bout of exercise, but the consequences of transient generation of signal X may persist well beyond the period of tonic contractile activity. Furthermore, if the kinetics of any step in the pathway triggered by signal X are slow, as might be expected if new protein synthesis of a regulatory factor is required, then a considerable time may elapse between the generation of signal X and its ultimate response (increased transcription of a specific gene encoding a protein of oxidative metabolism).

Experimental Approaches to Identification of Signal X and of Regulatory Pathways Triggered by Signal X

One strategy to identify signal X or components of pathways that are triggered by signal X is to attempt to reproduce or to inhibit the effects of contractile activity on specific genes by pharmacological manipulation of muscle cells in culture or in experimental animals. A limited number of experiments of this type have suggested that cAMP or calcium ion may be involved in the regulation of genes encoding proteins of oxidative metabolism. Intramuscular concentrations of both cAMP and calcium appear to be augmented during muscle contractions in vivo (Kraus, Bernard, & Williams, 1988; Streter, Lopez, Alamo, Mabuchi, & Gergely, 1987), and treatment of cultured skeletal myotubes with drugs that elevate cAMP and/or calcium promote increased synthesis of proteins of oxidative metabolism (Freerksen, Schroedl, Johnson, & Hartzell, 1986; Kagan & Freedman, 1974; Lawrence & Salsgiver, 1984; Sullivan et al., 1985; Liang et al., 1979). Despite many potential pitfalls, further experimentation of this type would appear to be a productive avenue.

A second and potentially more definitive strategy for elucidating pathways responsible for regulation of gene expression by contractile activity in muscle begins with the biochemical characterization of *trans-*

activator proteins that regulate genes that encode proteins of oxidative metabolism. Experimental techniques to accomplish this task are now available (Kadonaga & Tjian, 1986; Reinberg, Horikoshi, & Roeder, 1987) and have been spectacularly successful when applied to other important problems of gene regulation. Although this approach has promise, several special problems currently limit the application of advanced molecular biological methods to the study of gene regulation by contractile activity in muscle. First, there is as yet no adequate model system by which the investigator can induce effects in cultured myocytes that faithfully reproduce those evoked by exercise conditioning of intact muscles. The absence of an adequate cell culture model severely limits the types of molecular biological studies that can be performed. It remains to be determined whether this problem can be solved by technical innovations, or whether critical conditions necessary for this response simply cannot be reproduced in cultured cells.

In vitro transcription assays have been used successfully to identify *trans*-activator proteins in nuclear extracts prepared from intact tissues (e.g., liver) of experimental animals (Gorski, Carmeiro, & Schibler, 1986). If similar methods could be applied to extracts of muscle tissues, then well-characterized animal models of the effects of tonic contractile activity on skeletal muscle could be employed for studies of transcriptional regulation. This approach has some promise, but will be hampered by the special difficulties associated with cell fractionation of adult striated muscle tissues. Furthermore, interpretation of the results of in vitro transcription assays is sometimes difficult, because such results may be incompatible with important features of gene regulation in vivo (Sen & Baltimore, 1987).

Summary

I have presented a theoretical framework for consideration of a question that is central to the study of exercise: By what mechanisms do skeletal muscle fibers sense and respond to a change in tonic contractile activity by increasing their capacity to provide energy by oxidative metabolism? I suggest that this question can be considered as a problem of gene regulation and that emerging techniques of molecular biology create opportunities for testing specific hypotheses germane to this question. Although many difficulties associated with this approach can be identified, the importance of the question and the increasing power of the experimental techniques that can be brought to bear on this problem make this area an exciting frontier of exercise research.

References

Arndt, K., & Fink, E.R. (1986). GCN4 protein, a positive transcription factor in yeast, binds general control promoters at all 5' TGACTC

3′ sequences. *Proceedings of the National Academy of Science USA,* **83,** 8516–8520.

Booth, F.W., & Watson, P.A. (1985). Control of adaptations in protein levels in response to exercise. *Federation Proceedings,* **44,** 2293–2300.

Celenza, J.L., & Carlson, M. (1986). A yeast gene that is essential for release from glucose repression encodes a protein kinase. *Science,* **233,** 1175–1180.

Freerksen, D.L., Schroedl, N.A., Johnson, G.V.W., & Hartzell, C.R. (1986). Increased aerobic glucose oxidation by cAMP in cultured regenerated skeletal myotubes. *American Journal of Physiology,* **250,** C713–C719.

Galbo, H. (1983). *Hormonal and metabolic adaptation to exercise.* New York: Thieme–Stratton.

Gorski, K., Carmeiro, M., & Schibler, U. (1986). Tissue-specific *in vitro* transcription from the mouse albumin promoter. *Cell,* **47,** 767–776.

Guarente, L. & Mason, T. (1983). Heme regulates transcription of the CYC1 gene of S. cerevesiae via an upstream activation site. *Cell,* **32,** 1279–1286.

Henriksson, J., Chi, M.M-Y., Hintz, S., Young, D.A., Kaiser, K.K., Salmons, S. & Lowry, O.H. (1986). Chronic stimulation of mammalian muscle: Changes in enzymes of six metabolic pathways. *American Journal of Physiology,* **251,** C614–C632.

Henriksson, J., Galbo, H., & Blomstrand, E. (1982). Role of the motor nerve in activity-induced enzymatic adaptation in skeletal muscle. *American Journal of Physiology,* **242,** C272–C277.

Holloszy, J.O., & Coyle, E.F. (1984). Adaptations of skeletal muscle to endurance exercise and their metabolic consequences. *Journal of Applied Physiology,* **56,** 831–838.

Hoppeler, H., Howald, H., Conley, K., Lindstedt, S.L., Claassen, H., Vock, P., & Weibel, E.R. (1985). Endurance training in humans: Aerobic capacity and structure of skeletal muscle. *Journal of Applied Physiology,* **59,** 320–327.

Ji, L.L., Lennon, D.L.F., Kochan, R.G., Nagle, J.F., & Lardy, H.A. (1986). Enzymatic adaptation to physical training under β-blockade in the rat: Evidence of a β_2-adrenergic mechanism in skeletal muscle. *Journal of Clinical Investigation,* **78,** 771–778.

Johnston, S.A., Zavortink, M.J., Debouck, C., & Hopper, J.E. (1986). Functional domains of the yeast regulatory protein GAL4. *Proceedings of the National Academy of Sciences of the United States of America,* **83,** 6553–6557.

Kadonaga, J.T., & Tjian, R. (1986). Affinity purification of sequence-specific DNA binding proteins. *Proceedings of the National Academy of Sciences of the United States of America,* **83,** 5889–5893.

Kagan, L.J., & Freedman, A. (1974). Studies on the effects of acetylcholine, epinephrine, dibutyryl cyclic adenosine monophosphate, theophylline, and calcium on the synthesis of myoglobin in muscle cell cultures estimated by radioimmunoassay. *Experimental Cell Research,* **88,** 135–142.

Kraus, W.E., Bernard, T.S. & Williams, R.S. (1988). A possible role of cAMP in regulation of gene expression by contractile activity in muscle. *Clinical Research,* **36,** 542a.

Lawrence, J.C., Jr., & Salsgiver, W.J. (1984). Evidence that levels of malate dehydrogenase and fumarase are increased by cAMP in rat myotubes. *American Journal of Physiology,* **247,** C33–C38.

Liang, C.S., Tuttle, R.R., Hood, W.B., & Haralambos, G. (1979). Conditioning effects of chronic infusions of dobutamine: Comparison with exercise training. *Journal of Clinical Investigation,* **64,** 613–619.

Pette, D. (1984). Activity-induced fast to slow transitions in mammalian muscle. *Medicine and Science in Sports and Exercise,* **16,** 517–528.

Pette, D., & Vrbova, G. (1985). Neural control of phenotypic expression in mammalian muscle fibers. *Muscle & Nerve,* **8,** 676–689.

Pluskal, M.G., & Streter, F.A. (1983). Correlation between protein phenotype and gene expression in adult rabbit fast twitch muscles undergoing a fast to slow fiber transformation in response to electrical stimulation *in vivo. Biochemical and Biophysical Research Communications,* **113,** 325–331.

Reinberg, D., Horikoshi, M.I., & Roeder, R.G. (1987). Factors involved in specific transcription in mammalian RNA polymerase II. *Journal of Biological Chemistry,* **262,** 3322–3330.

Salmons, S., & Henriksson, J. (1981). The adaptive response of skeletal muscle to increased use. *Muscle & Nerve,* **4,** 94–105.

Saltin, B., & Gollnick, P.D. (1983). Skeletal muscle adaptability: Significance for metabolism and performance. In L.D.D. Peachey (Ed.), *Handbook of Physiology: Skeletal Muscle* (pp. 555–632). Bethesda, MD: American Physiological Society.

Seedorf, U., Leberer, E., Kirschbaum, B.J., & Pette, D. (1986). Neural control of gene expression in skeletal muscle: Effects of chronic stimulation on lactate dehydrogenase isoenzymes and citrate synthase. *Biochemical Journal,* **239,** 115–120.

Sen, R., & Baltimore, D. (1987). In vitro transcription of immunoglobulin genes in a B-cell extract: Effects of enhancer and promoter sequences. *Molecular and Cellular Biology,* **7** 1989–1994.

Streter, F.A., Lopez, J.R., Alamo, L., Mabuchi, K., & Gergely, J. (1987). Changes in intracellular ionized Ca concentration associated with muscle fiber type transformation. *American Journal of Physiology,* **253,** C296–C300.

Sullivan, M.J., Binkley, P.F., Unverferth, D.V., Ren, J., Boudoulas, H., Bashore, T.M., Merola, A.J., & Leier, C.V. (1985). Prevention of bedrest-induced physical deconditioning by daily dobutamine infusions: Implications for drug-induced physical conditioning. *Journal of Clinical Investigation,* **76,** 1632–1642.

Underwood, L.E., & Williams, R.S. (1987). Pretranslational regulation of myoglobin gene expression. *American Journal of Physiology,* **252,** C450–C453.

Williams, R.S., Garcia-Moll, M., Mellor, J., Salmons, S., & Harlan, W. (1987). Adaptation of skeletal muscle to increased contractile activity. *Journal of Biological Chemistry,* **262,** 2764–2767.

Williams, R.S., Salmons, S., Newsholme, E.A., Kaufman, R.E., & Mellor, J. (1986). Regulation of nuclear and mitochondrial gene expression by contractile activity in skeletal muscle. *Journal of Biological Chemistry*, **261**, 376–380.

Wolfel, E.E., Hiatt, W.R., Brammell, H.L. Carry, M.R., Ringel, S.P., Travis, V., & Horwitz, L.D. (1986). Effects of selective and nonselective β-adrenergic blockade on mechanisms of exercise conditioning. *Circulation*, **74**, 664–674.

Xitomer, R.S., Sellers, J.W., McCarter, D.W., Hastings, G.A., Wick, P., & Lowry, C.V. (1987). Elements involved in oxygen regulation of the Saccharomyces cerevesiae CyC7 Gene. *Molecular and Cellular Biology*, **7**, 2212–2220.

Part III

A Corporate Perspective

What Is the Justification for the Establishment of a Corporate Fitness Program?

Edward J. Bernacki

Tenneco Incorporated
Houston, Texas

Fitness programs in industry have been associated with reduced health care costs, decreased absenteeism, and increased productivity. Although it is unclear whether fitness center use induces these beneficial work behaviors, there is evidence that they are more prevalent among exercising employees and that they predate exercise adherence. Consequently, fitness programs are valuable to corporations because of their ability to attract and retain persons with beneficial work behaviors, and this utility commences at the time of program initiation. Furthermore, there is little evidence to indicate that participants in these programs have increased injury rates or medical care costs.

The primary aim of a corporation is to generate profits and increase assets for shareholders. Secondary goals are to provide employment and to increase the material wealth of the society in which a corporation operates. A high priority is placed on achieving the first objective, and although the secondary goals are deemed beneficial they are understandably of lower priority. It goes without saying that fitness programs do not directly increase corporate profits or assets. How then are they justified by corporate managers? Driver and Ratliff (1982) postulate that managers perceive exercise as reducing health care claims and absenteeism by reducing the incidence of illness. Managers also feel that physical fitness programs, by increasing organizational cohesiveness or satisfaction with the corporation, lead to desirable work behaviors (e.g., increased productivity, decreased turnover, decreased absenteeism). This in turn increases profitability and the perception that the corporation is a socially responsible one committed to the well-being of its employees.

Are there data to support these perceptions? It has been well demonstrated that increased exercise activity is strongly associated with a reduction in cardiovascular disease risk factors (Fox, Naughton, & Haskell, 1971; Paffenbarger, Wing, & Hyde, 1983) as well as a reduction in morbidity and mortality from heart disease (Paffenbarger, Hyde, Wing,

151

& Hsieh, 1986; Peters, Cody, & Bischoff, 1983). Given that employers in the United States, through disability and group health insurance policies, pay almost the full share of their employees' absenteeism and health care costs, any reduction in these expenses would reduce operating costs. Obviously, it takes years for lifestyle changes to have any effect on reducing morbidity and illness costs. Will time permit a corporation to benefit from good health habits such as exercise among its employees? In almost all instances, although initial results have been positive, studies extended over longer periods (Bowne, Russell, Morgan, Optenberg, & Clarke, 1984; Shephard, 1985; Song, Shephard, & Cox, 1982) have been unable to demonstrate the beneficial effects of exercise due to high employee turnover and cessation of exercise among those studied. Therefore, a good case has not and probably never will be made for supporting corporate exercise programs based on the physiologic benefits of exercise.

It may not be necessary, however, to demonstrate a long-term effect of exercise to justify programs. Rather, they may be supported by the fact that exercisers possess attributes independent of exercise that are beneficial to a corporation. There is evidence that, in the short term, participants in an exercise program are absent less often and require fewer health services than their nonexercising colleagues (Bowne et al., 1984; Cox, Shephard, & Corey, 1981). In a study of job performance and exercise, Bernacki and Baun (1984) found that a significantly greater proportion of exercisers were high performers than were nonexercisers and that this attribute predated exercise adherence. Likewise, the same authors noted that exercisers had lower health care costs, absenteeism (Baun, Bernacki, & Tsai, 1986), and turnover (Tsai, Baun, & Bernacki, 1987) and that this relationship was found at the start of a corporate fitness program, long before one could expect the beneficial effects of exercise on absenteeism or the cost of treating illnesses. White, Powell, Hogelin, Gentry, and Formum (1987) have shown that individuals who smoke less, wear seatbelts, and are not obese are more likely than those who do not to exercise at a rate higher than 3 kcal per kg per day in their leisure time. Thus, it appears that current exercisers have many attributes that are beneficial to a corporation, and that their presence in the work force is desirable.

Although it is indeed difficult to find data justifying exercise programs, there is a tendency on the part of some researchers (Bowne et al., 1984; Cox et al., 1981) to extend the positive attributes of exercisers to those currently not exercising, overstating the case for exercise. These authors imply that if nonexercisers were induced to exercise, the magnitude of benefits to a corporation would be increased. In a study already alluded to, Bernacki and Baun (1984) found that performance levels among low-level exercisers were similar to those of nonexercisers. The implication of this finding is that a positive attribute of exercisers, high performance, is weakly or not at all associated with occasional or low-level exercisers. It suggests that there will be few short-term financial gains if sedentary individuals become occasional exercisers. Therefore, any savings that are attributed to exercisers probably should be limited to that segment of the working population alone and not be applied to nonexercisers. Above and beyond this, it is considerably easier and less expensive to provide facilities for dedicated exercisers than to induce nonexercisers to become exercisers, always a difficult (though worthy) task.

What does all this mean? It appears that the managers' perceptions of the benefits of an exercise program cited by Driver and Ratliff (1982) are on the whole correct—that fitness is associated with good performance and reduced medical costs and absenteeism. However, this is primarily due to attributes of exercisers and is not secondary to the beneficial effects of exercise. Because individuals choose to work for a particular corporation, the provision of an exercise facility by a company will increase the probability that highly motivated persons will select the company, increasing their representation in the work force. Eventually, if turnover rates are lower for exercisers (and we think this is the case), the exercising population will comprise a larger part of the work force. If it is large enough, the savings associated with exercise could have an impact on corporate profitability.

What are the negatives? Tsai, Bernacki, and Baun (1988) looked at the risks and costs of injury among participants of an employee fitness program. They found that injury rates and costs were virtually the same among participants and nonparticipants of the program. Others have shown higher injury rates among persons who engage in exercise (Koplan, Powell, Sikes, Shirley, & Campbell, 1982; Koplan, Siscovick, & Goldvaum, 1985; Walter, Sutton, McIntosh, & Connolly, 1985). The discrepancy lies in the amount and type of exercise that is related to injury. In a study by Tsai et al. (1988), corporate exercisers expended approximately 300 to 400 kcal per (low intensity) exercise session, whereas the other studies examined participants in contact sports or long distance running (high intensity exercise with a greater risk of injury).

What about expenses? The most significant costs of a fitness program are the capital costs related to building or renovating a facility for exercise use. These costs, of course, can be extremely high. In my experience, small, rather modest facilities can be constructed at low cost. Although these small facilities might not be an inducement for marginal or nonexercisers to engage in exercise, they will be for dedicated exercisers (individuals most likely to have a positive lifestyle and therefore most likely to benefit a corporation).

Operating costs of more corporate fitness facilities are low compared to private or public fitness clubs. At Tenneco Inc., costs range between $36 and $350 per member per year (Baun & Bernacki, 1987) to operate the company's 15 fitness centers. Low-end costs are associated with the smaller facilities (containing showers, lockers, and training equipment only), whereas the highest cost is related to the company's largest facility, which employs multiple staff members and contains a running track, racquetball courts, and exercise equipment (Bernacki & Baun, 1984).

From what I have seen and presented, there is very little to indicate that fitness programs will not benefit most corporations. Although I am admittedly biased, I truly feel that the strategy of enlightened U.S. businesses should be the design of fitness programs and facilities to attract and retain dedicated exercisers.

References

Baun, W.B., & Bernacki, E.J., (1987). Who are the corporate exercisers and what motivates them? In R.K. Dishman (Ed.), *Exercise adherence: Its impact on public health* (pp. 321–348). Champaign, IL: Human Kinetics.

Baun, W.B., Bernacki, E.J., & Tsai, S.P. (1986). A preliminary investigation: Effect of a corporate fitness program on absenteeism and health care cost. *Journal of Occupational Medicine, 28,* 18–22.

Bernacki, E.J., & Baun, W.B. (1984). The relationship of job performance to exercise adherence in a corporate fitness program. *Journal of Occupational Medicine, 26,* 229–231.

Bowne, D.W., Russell, M.L., Morgan, J.L., Optenberg, R.N., & Clarke, A.E. (1984). Reduced disability and health care costs in an industrial fitness program. *Journal of Occupational Medicine, 26,* 809–816.

Cox, M., Shephard, R.J., & Corey, P. (1981). Influence of an employee fitness programme upon fitness, productivity and absenteeism. *Ergonomics, 24,* 795–806.

Driver, R.W., & Ratliff, R.A. (1982). Employers' perceptions of benefits accrued from physical fitness programs. *Personnel Administrator,* August 21–26.

Fox, S.M., Naughton, I.P., & Haskell, W.L. (1971). Physical activity and the prevention of coronary heart disease. *Annals of Clinical Research, 3,* 404–432.

Koplan, J.P., Powell, K.E., Sikes, R.K., Shirley, R.W., & Campbell, C.C. (1982). An epidemiologic study of the benefits and risks of running. *Journal of the American Medical Association, 248,* 3118–3121.

Koplan, J.P., Siscovick, D.S., & Goldvaum, G.M. (1985). The risks of exercise: A public health view in injuries and hazards. *Public Health Reports, 100,* 189–195.

Paffenbarger, R.S., Hyde, R.T., Wing, A.L. & Hsieh, C. (1986). Physical activity, all-cause mortality, and longevity of college alumni. *New England Journal of Medicine, 314,* 605–614.

Paffenbarger, R.S., Wing, R.T., & Hyde, R.T. (1983). Physical activity and the incidence of hypertension in college alumni. *American Journal of Epidemiology, 117,* 245–257.

Peters, R.K., Cody, L.D., & Bischoff, D.P. (1983). Physical fitness and subsequent myocardial infarction in healthy workers. *Journal of the American Medical Association, 249,* 3052–3056.

Shephard, R.J. (1985). The impact of exercise upon medical costs. *Sports Medicine, 2,* 133–143.

Song, T.K., Shephard, R.J., & Cox, M. (1982). Absenteeism, employee turnover and sustained exercise participation. *Journal of Sports Medicine, 22*, 391–399.

Tsai, S.P., Baun, W.B., & Bernacki, E.J. (1987). The relationship of employee turnover to exercise adherence in a corporate fitness program. *Journal of Occupational Medicine, 29.*

Tsai, S.P., Bernacki, E.J., & Baun, W.B. (1988). Injury prevalence and associated costs among participants of an employee fitness program. *Preventive Medicine, 17*, 475–482.

Walter, S.D., Sutton, J.R., McIntosh, H.M., & Connolly, C. (1985). The etiology of sports injuries: A review of methodologies. *Sports Medicine, 2*, 47–58.

White, C.C., Powell, E.K., Hogelin, G.C., Gentry, M.M, & Formum, M.R. (1987). The behavioral risk factor surveys: IV. The descriptive epidemiology of exercise. *American Journal of Preventive Medicine, 3*, 304–310.

The Coors Wellness Process

Max L. Morton
Coors Wellness Center, Golden, Colorado

The Adolph Coors Company was founded more than 100 years ago by Adolph Herman Joseph Coors. Today his grandson and great-grandsons are still producing fine beers in the same Golden, Colorado, location. The Company employs 10,500 people internationally, with 6,500 located in Golden. The work force is divided into 52% salaried nonexempt and 48% salaried exempt. The average age of the work force is 44 years.

The following quote from "Our Values" is the foundation of our successful wellness program: "These values can only be fulfilled by quality people dedicated to quality relationships within our Company. We foster personal and professional growth and development and encourage wellness in body, mind, and spirit for all employees" (Adolph Coors Company Board of Directors, 1986).

A History of Wellness at Coors

Good health and well-being among Coors employees has been an important aspect of the company from its beginning. Our comprehensive recreation program began with softball games, company picnics, and other social events soon after the company started. The Adolph Coors Company has had a policy of no smoking in the workplace, except in designated lunchroom areas, for over 20 years.

In the late 1960s, the Coors Medical Center opened to meet the needs of employees with on-the-job injuries and illnesses. In the 1970s, an employee assistance program began and was soon expanded to employee and family counseling services. Today employees and dependents receive occupational injury and mental health diagnostic and referral services free of charge.

William K. Coors, chairman of the board of the Adolph Coors Company, was and still is the leader of the company wellness movement. He believes the company has a moral obligation to develop and maintain a work environment that encourages every employee to be dedicated to

157

wellness. In addition, wellness is an integral part of the Coors management style. Accordingly, in 1981 the 25,000-square-foot Coors Wellness Center opened in a renovated supermarket at the main entrance of the brewery.

Our Mission Statement

The mission of the Wellness Center is to increase employees' and their families' awareness and knowledge of healthy lifestyles, to provide incentives and programs to enable lifestyle changes, and to support and maintain employees' and their families' self-actions in healthy lifestyles. Because wellness depends on individual lifestyle, the Coors Wellness Program is designed to encourage habits and lifestyles that affect wellness and to provide programs that encourage behavior changes to improve general health and well-being. In recognition that one of the greatest influences on individual lifestyle change is the immediate family, the Wellness Program includes retirees, spouses, and dependents 12 years of age or older.

The Social Marketing Model

All wellness programs are designed to follow a social marketing model described by Philip Kotler that includes the following elements:

- Awareness: The existence of a problem must be established.
- Education: An educational program must present information, in layperson's terms, that makes the issues interesting and understandable.
- Incentives: Change is more likely when individuals perceive clearly the personal and social benefits of change.
- Programs: It is necessary to provide skill training in how to start to make changes by providing step-by-step, "how-to" programs.
- Self-action: This strategy enables individuals to take specific actions to adopt new behaviors.
- Maintenance: Inputs are required to provide a sense of social support and approval for changed behaviors.

The Wellness Process is divided into six different program areas or modules: health hazard appraisal and screening; smoking cessation; physical fitness; nutrition; stress management; and slimness. In some situations both primary and secondary prevention modules are provided. Each of the modules with results (where available) is described here.

Coors Health Hazard Appraisal (HHA)

The Coors Health Hazard Appraisal (HHA) was initiated in 1984 as an awareness and education program for Coors employees and spouses living anywhere in the United States. A health insurance co-pay shift of 5% additional coverage was provided for individuals completing the questionnaire and meeting criterion A of +1.9 years or less difference in chronological age (CA)/health age (HA), termed "not-at-risk" (NAR); or criterion B of +2.0 years or more difference in CA/HA, termed "at-risk" (AR) and receiving interpretive information by one-to-one contact or by phone or mail. By the end of 1984, 8,400 eligible individuals (60%) were enrolled; by the end of 1987, 11,000 (80%). In response to the total group profile, Coors has initiated on-site mammography, a company-wide seat belt campaign, on-site cholesterol measurement, a company-wide blood pressure education campaign, and blood pressure machine placement throughout production and office areas. "Repeat" appraisals completed in 1987 by 418 (59%) of the 1984 AR employees resulted in 72% now NAR and 28% still AR, but a total group improvement in HA estimated at $331 per person in annual health cost reduction. The average annual program costs are $5 per enrollee, which includes a contract half-time educator/administrator.

The Wellness Plus Program

The primary objective of Wellness Plus was to offer a simple, broad-based health awareness program to encourage more employees to pursue healthier lifestyles. The main purpose was to appeal to those employees who had not taken advantage of the wellness programs already offered. The program consisted of a simple questionnaire, strong management support, gentle peer pressure, nominal incentives, and competition. The areas covered on the questionnaire were cholesterol levels, blood pressure, smoking, nutrition, exercise, lifestyle habits (such as seat belt, moderate consumption of alcohol, flossing teeth), mental health/stress, and regular medical and dental care. Each question was assigned points according to its overall impact on health. Average points were determined for each department on a quarterly basis. Interdepartmental and divisional competition kept interest in the program high and contributed greatly to its success. The program was piloted in the sales and marketing department in 1986. Due to the success of the pilot program it was expanded to the rest of the Adolph Coors Company in 1987. Seventy-three percent of employees (4,157) in the departments involved participated, and 38% (1,503) reported positive modification of their lifestyle.

Wellness Center Medical Screening

The Coors Wellness Center uses a medical screening questionnaire for every participant in the physical fitness module. The questions focus on coronary artery disease risk factors, hypertension, smoking, elevated cholesterol, family history, diabetes, chest and leg pain history, medications, and orthopedic injury history. Participants are identified in high-, moderate- and low-risk categories and are referred for further evaluation and/ or other modules of the wellness program.

Included in the Wellness Center's evaluations are cholesterol screening, percent body fat measurements (skinfold caliper method), and one-to-one education sessions regarding proper use of exercise equipment. Educating users about safe, effective forms of exercise and tailoring exercise programs to fit individual needs are emphasized by the Wellness Center staff.

Treadmill Screening

From the inception of the Wellness Center, graded exercise tests have been used to screen some participants prior to initiating an exercise program. The majority of tests have been submaximal studies to 85% of the subject's age-corrected estimated maximal heart rate. Indications for a submaximal exercise evaluation include resting systolic blood pressure greater than 140 mm/Hg, resting diastolic blood pressure greater than 90 mm/Hg, medication for elevated blood pressure, age of 35 years or older with several coronary artery disease risk factors, and requests for exercise program guidelines. A few participants undergo a 12-lead symptom-limited maximal stress test with the Wellness Center's cardiologist. Indications for a maximal stress test include known coronary disease (myocardial infarction, coronary artery bypass graph (CABG), post precutaneous transluminal coronary angioplasty (PTCA), abnormal ST changes); known or suspected peripheral vascular disease; systolic blood pressure greater than 250 mm/Hg or diastolic blood pressure greater than 110 mm/Hg on a submaximal evaluation; insulin-dependent diabetes and age 30 years or more or diabetes for more than 6 years; evaluation of suspicious chest pain; entrance into modification programs; request of the participant's personal doctor; request of the Coors Medical Center. A maximal stress test may be part of an employee's annual physical exam. In addition, the Coors Medical Center may require a symptom-limited maximal treadmill to certify employees to wear Scott Air Packs (an industrial respirator).

The cost to Coors in 1987 for maximal exercise tests was $43,148. If the tests had been obtained in the community, the estimated cost would have been $154,770. Thus, maximal exercise evaluations have provided a significant savings to Coors Industries while providing a timely service to the employees and staff of the Wellness and Medical Center.

Cholesterol and Blood Pressure Screening

Serum cholesterol levels have received a great deal of attention from both medical scientists and the media. Cholesterol level is a major risk factor in coronary artery disease. For each percentage point cholesterol is reduced, risks decrease twofold. To facilitate cholesterol awareness and education a Kodak DT60 Analyzer was purchased. In 1987 over 2,000 individuals were screened and educated about cholesterol (see Table 1).

Table 1   Numbers of Individuals and Costs to the Company of Cholesterol Screening

Number	Cholesterol (mg/dl)	Cost/test
40	>300	$2 (Our cost)
227	251–300	$6 (Outside cost)
754	201–250	
990	≤ 200	$4 (Savings)

Blood Pressure Screening

Employees and spouses of Coors can get their blood pressure checked at the Wellness Center or the Medical Center by a staff member or at one of seven automatic blood pressure machines located throughout the production and work areas. Five of these machines are at fixed locations, and two machines are rotated on a regular schedule. In a typical month 5,000 to 6,000 tests are recorded on the machines. Educational materials and consultation for high blood pressure are available at the Coors Wellness Center and Coors Medical Center.

Coorscreen

An on-site breast cancer screening program, Coorscreen, was instituted by the company in September 1985. The purposes of the program were (a) to create an ongoing awareness of breast cancer for all female employees and spouses and (b) to lower company health care costs through early detection of breast cancer. Eligible women included those 35 and over, those not pregnant, and those not screened within the past year. Coors corporate communications, Medical Center and Wellness Center staffs have worked cooperatively to insure ongoing participation.

To date over 2,300 women have been screened (71% of all eligible employees and 40% of spouses). Eligibility included 4,076 women. Of those screened, there have been over 200 abnormal screenings, and four early malignancies were detected. An early stage breast cancer costs Coors approximately $18,000, while a late stage cancer costs $60,000. To date the program costs are $63,628, including screenings at $55 each ($40 covered by Coors), needle aspirations, and other necessary tests. The estimated costs to Coors if the cancers detected at early stages had advanced to metastatic disease were $289,000. This figure is based on direct medical costs, short-term disability costs, and personnel costs. An estimated cost effectiveness figure in dollars saved for Coors would be $225,372. The cost effectiveness for doing on-site screenings is also important. Metro Denver mammography costs average $100. Screening would have cost $230,000 to do on the outside, while on-site screening costs totaled $63,628, for a savings of $166,372. The cost effectiveness in terms of human lives is immeasurable.

Exercise Programs

Employees, spouses, and dependents (age 12 and over) are eligible to utilize exercise programs at the Coors Wellness Center after clearance of a medical history form. Submaximal and maximal stress tests are administered for those who request exercise prescriptions or who demonstrate significant risk factors. Individuals may exercise on their own or take a variety of classes. Group class activities concentrate on cardiovascular fitness, with 13 classes offered daily.

Toning and strength classes are also available. Special populations offered group classes are senior retirees and spouses of employees, obese individuals, ski fitness enthusiasts, and those with cardiac disease. Equipment, facilities, and additional services include an 1/8-mile indoor track, treadmills, stationary cycles, rowing machines, jogging tramps, and strength equipment.

Nutrition Education

The nutrition education activities at Coors focus on practical issues that affect making healthy food choices. Cooking classes and tasting parties introduce employees to nutritious foods and cooking techniques. Grocery store shopping tours and practice at reading labels challenge participants to compare the nutrient density of foods and select the best brands. Slim Livin' classes meet weekly to investigate ways to blend exercise and good eating habits with a busy lifestyle. Nutrition traymats for cafeteria trays that reach all Coors employees contain a simplified nutrition message and easy recipes. Healthy foods are designated in employee cafeterias as "Treat Yourself Right" items to assist employees in making good nutritional decisions.

A priority for nutrition efforts at Coors is using a variety of delivery methods. Classes, articles in the corporate newspaper, informational traymats, posters, and brown bag lunch seminars are various cost-effective ways that Coors delivers nutrition messages. Employees with specific dietary concerns can schedule a consultation with a registered dietitian, although most weight-loss and cardiovascular health questions can be answered in scheduled classes. Spouses are strongly encouraged to attend all nutrition activities because their support is invaluable to the behavior change process.

Stress Management Services

Coors stress management services consist of three programs. One addresses general stress management in eight 1-hr weekly small group sessions (7–15 participants). The first session provides an overview of stress and stress management and gives homework focusing on heightened awareness of personal stressors and stress responses (cognitive, imagery, emotional, physiological, and behavioral components). The next six sessions stress enhancing environmental change strategies (e.g., directly altering sources of stress) and behavioral skills (e.g., assertiveness, cognitive, rational, task-oriented, problem-solving, relaxation, breathing-cured relaxation, and coping skills). Because of the wider applicability, greater attention is given to relaxation and cognitive coping skills that are taught through a combination of anxiety management training and stress inoculation training. The final session, 7 weeks after the seventh session, serves review and maintenance functions.

Eighty-two of 97 participants (15 had incomplete data) in the last 2 years completed two Stress Situation measures (0–100 rating of stress in the two worst ongoing stress situations) and two Stress Symptom measures (0–100 rating of the two strongest indices of stress-related physiological arousal), one Trait Anxiety Inventory, and one Trait Anger Scale on a pre-post program basis. A multivariate, repeated measures analysis of variance revealed a significant overall change from pre- to postassessment (F [6, 76] = 75.80, p < .001). Univariate analyses revealed significant reductions of personal-situational stress reactions, stress-related physiological arousal, general anxiety, and general anger.

The second stress management class is a general relaxation program of four 1-hr weekly small group sessions. Each meeting introduces a new method of relaxation—progressive relaxation, relaxation without tension, imagery-based relaxation, and autogenic relaxation.

Participants are trained in each method during the session and between sessions use a manual and four audio cassettes to repeat the training in one or more tape segments. Initial reports indicate attainment of relaxation within sessions, moderate regular use of tapes, and general stress and tension reduction.

The third class is a program on anger management, consisting of eight 90-min weekly small group sessions. The class focuses on (a) increased awareness of anger responses and provoking situations; (b) relaxation coping skills for control of emotional and physiological arousal; (c) cognitive restructuring and problem-solving skills for control of anger-engendering thoughts; and (d) behavioral change strategies, especially empathic listening, assertiveness, and interpersonal negotiation, for altered interpersonal reactions. The program is a combination of the cognitive-relaxation and social skills approaches. A pre-post evaluation revealed reductions in situational anger, general anger, anger-related physiological arousal, and general anxiety.

Smart Heart

Next to low back pain, coronary artery disease is the second costliest medical problem among Coors employees. Smart Heart is a systematic effort at primary prevention of coronary disease involving both risk identification and risk modification programs. The Smart Heart risk modification program meets 5 days per week for 6 weeks. The program includes 1 hr each day of supervised aerobic exercise and 1 hr of education for a total of 60 contact hr. The education classes emphasize nutrition, wellness principles, and self-responsibility. All the classes increase the likelihood that the participants will assume responsibility for their own health behaviors upon completion of the program. Evaluations completed at entry and exit include a lipid profile comprised of total cholesterol, LDL-C, HDL-C, triglycerides, ApoA-1, and Apo-B; glucose; resting blood pressure; smoking history; body weight; body composition; and aerobic capacity via a 12-lead maximal stress test.

Preliminary results of the Smart Heart program show significant changes ($p < .05$) pre- and postparticipation in body weight, body composition, systolic blood pressure, diastolic blood pressure, aerobic capacity, total cholesterol, LDL-C, and glucose. Six-month followup data continue to show similar trends. The program has not yet completed its first full year of operation, and thus it is premature to speculate about the potential cost savings to Coors. Future plans include continued modification of the program content and structure. It needs to have frequent start dates and to be equally convenient to all Coors employees.

Parenting Modules

The purpose of the Coors parenting modules is to enhance parenting skills and to enable healthy family interactions. The program consists of four 90-min sessions. Material presented is drawn from various sources, including the work of Haim Ginott, Thomas Gordon, Eric Erikson, and Rudolph Dreikurs. Programs focus on these topics: Adolescents: Who Are They and Why Do They Do What They Do?; Problems Parents Face; Developmental Appropriateness: What's Normal for Teens; Characteristics and Motivators; Assertive Discipline Techniques for Parents of Teens; Parenting Skills: Tips for Making It Through; Parenting the Adolescent in the New Age; Dealing with Drugs, Sex, and Rock n' Roll; and single parenting skills.

LIFESTEPS: Weight Management

"How can I manage my weight?" is the most frequently asked nutrition-related question at Coors. In selecting a program to address this need, Coors looked for something that was educationally sound and focused on both good nutrition and exercise. The LIFESTEPS: Weight Management program, developed by the National Dairy Council, was selected because it emphasizes life-long, step-by-step behavior changes in physical activity and eating habits. Classes are team-taught by a registered dietitian and an exercise specialist. In 15 weeks, participants develop an individualized eating and exercise plan; no "diet" is given.

Surveys of past LIFESTEPS participants have been encouraging. Average weight loss through the course of the program is 1 to 2 lb per week. One year after completing the program, 48% have continued to lose weight or maintain weight loss, and 55% report exercising at least 3 to 4 times per week. Reported long-term dietary changes include eating a better variety of foods, increasing consumption of fruits and vegetables, selecting lower-calorie items for home and when eating out, and eating smaller portion sizes.

Smoking Cessation

The Adolph Coors Company is committed to a smoke-free workplace. The present smoking management class format has been offered for the past 3 years. Coors treats smoking as a dangerous drug dependency. Smoking is comparable to heroin addiction in its sufferers' inability to quit. It is six times more addictive than alcohol. The program consists of 24 total classroom hours. Twenty of these are scheduled during the first 90 days of quitting. In addition, there are meetings at 6 months, 9 months, and 1 year postcessation.

Beginning with an information seminar, the program is outlined in detail. Not everyone interested is allowed to take the course. Anyone with a recent divorce, a death in the family, a major job loss, or current enrollment in an alcohol treatment or a weight loss program is generally considered under too much stress to simultaneously try to quit smoking. Coors smoking management classes teach the smoker how to avoid and eliminate smoking urges, how to lose the desire to smoke, how to make newly learned skills a part of a lifestyle and, very important, how to minimize weight gain.

Since 1985, 219 participants have enrolled in the program. In 1985, 35 smokers completed the program; 69% were still not smoking at 1 year. During 1986, 37 people completed the program; 75% were still not smoking at 1 year. In 1987, 103 people attended the program; 1-year followup data are not yet available. From an internal study, Coors estimates a $2 return on every $1 invested in its smoking management classes.

Prenatal Program

Coors developed a comprehensive prenatal awareness and education program in 1987. The program promotes healthy pregnancies and healthier babies, increases awareness of the causes of birth defects, promotes healthy lifestyles for parents, and increases the probability of reduced insurance costs.

Participants get prior maternity benefit approval from Coors Insurance. The treating physician and parents then must complete a screening for high-risk pregnancies as early as possible (before the first trimester), facilitating early referrals of high-risk cases. The Coors occupational health department educates prospective parents about possible hazards and exposures in the work environments. The Coors Wellness Center educates parents about the effects of smoking, diet, chemical use, lack of exercise, and infectious diseases, therefore promoting healthier babies.

Cardiac Rehabilitation

Cardiac rehabilitation became part of the Coors Wellness Center program in the fall of 1981, shortly after the center opened. Phase II, the early posthospitalization cardiac program, was developed from the premises that, first, rehabilitation is a wellness program for the employee with cardiovascular disease and, second, that it is appropriate for Coors, a self-insured company, to make a strong effort to reduce the costs related to heart disease.

To date 223 employees, spouses, or retired employees have participated in the program. Of the employees, 75% were salary nonexempt workers. Every effort is made to enroll the employee within 2 weeks of discharge from the hospital for a cardiac event. The 12-week program includes 36 exercise conditioning sessions, screening for psychosocial disability, stress management, nutrition, a 12-class comprehensive education program for the employee and spouse, and a strong vocational component. Early in the program, a job-site visit and thorough job assessment are performed by a Coors team vocational specialist. Job-specific muscle strengthening exercises are built into the exercise prescription.

When the Coors team feels that the employee is ready to return to work, a meeting is scheduled with the employee, the employee's supervisor, the program coordinator, the medical director, and often the vocational counselor. At this meeting, a phased return to work and any necessary job modifications are negotiated. The usual goal is to have the employee working full time (except for the 6 hr a week spent in the rehabilitation program) by the time the 12-week rehabilitation program is completed.

To date, 98% of these employees have returned to work, all of them to the job held prior to the cardiac event. In approximately 35,000 hours of Wellness Center contact with cardiac employees, including both Phase II and the Phase III maintenance program, there has been one death, which was not related to exercise. In the first 6 years of the program, savings to Coors have exceeded $1.6 million through wage savings and reduced program and exercise test costs. Potential savings in retraining costs and fewer employees on long-term disability following a cardiac event have been estimated. Coors cardiac rehabilitation in an industrial setting has proven to be feasible, safe, and cost-effective.

Orthopedic Rehabilitation

Rehabilitation of orthopedic sports-related injuries is monitored at the Coors Wellness Center. From the beginning of the program, having a staff member to provide programs for back and orthopedic problems was important. As work loads increased a certified athletic trainer was added. The athletic trainer provides injury evaluation and develops a rehabilitative protocol that can be performed at the Wellness Center.

The trainer is on site up to 9 hr a week, evaluating 8 to 10 people a week. Ten to 15% of initial evaluations are referred to a physician. The remaining 85% to 90% are placed on a protocol and are monitored on a weekly to biweekly basis. If no progress is made these individuals are also referred to a physician. The physician referral rate for this latter group is approximately 5%. Outside physicians also utilize the Wellness Center for rehabilitation of their Coors patients and family members, which results in a cost savings to Coors.

Back Program

Coors Well Back Program is a two-session course on back wellness and injury prevention. Employees attend two sessions and are instructed by physical therapists who specialize in spinal dysfunction. The course content consists of anatomy, the aggravation concept, activities of daily living, posture, body mechanics in lifting, return to normal activities, work and rest positions, first aid, and a comprehensive exercise program.

Class members participate in an obstacle course and a sample exercise program and ask questions. Any member not already participating in other wellness programs is encouraged to utilize those services in order to decrease back pain aggravation as it relates to smoking cessation, nutritional counseling, stress management, and exercise. The goal of the class is self-responsibility for back pain through self-awareness and lifestyle assessment or changes.

Less-Successful Modules and Areas

Not all Coors Wellness efforts have been "successful." Modules for alcohol and drug abuse prevention were not well received, and new strategies are being developed. Difficulties exist in delivering quality programs to remote-site employees. Salary nonexempt participation is lower than salary exempt. Special modules such as back and orthopedic rehabilitation and screening services near the work areas have demonstrated improved penetration of the wellness concept into the nonexempt employee population.

Measures of Economic Cost Impact

William K. Coors and the Coors board of directors believe that in-depth and scientific evaluation would double the cost of the Coors wellness effort. However, within existing resources some measurement has been done (see Table 2).

Table 2   The Economic Cost Impact of Coors Wellness Programs in 1987

Savings/program	Amount ($)
Area of savings	
Actual	1,844,609
Assumed	519,690
Total savings	2,364,299
Operational cost	
Wellness center	565,423
Well back and orthopedic rehabilitation	9,912
Stress management	14,100
Parenting	1,440
Mammography	42,840
Total cost	633,715
Total net economic cost impact	1,730,584
Return of investment ratio	3.73 : 1

The Coors Wellness Center is an effective lifestyle change program. Usage has increased 37% from 1981 to 1987, with over 117,000 uses of the Center's programs in 1987. Studies of health insurance costs indicate reductions of 13% for regular users of the Coors wellness programs. On-site cardiac rehabilitation and mammography are cost-effective and psychosocially effective. Well-designed programs in smoking cessation, weight loss, and stress management result in long-term desired changes. Coors' programs focus on quality of life issues and are individualized for all employees, retirees, and their families. The diseases that are lifestyle-related take 30 or more years to develop; therefore, logic and current cost-effectiveness trends encourage maintenance of high-quality work site wellness programs.

Health and Physical Fitness Programs:
Why They're Important to Business

J. Roger King
PepsiCo., Inc.
Purchase, New York

"You can't run a successful company with people only 'half well.' " Those words were said many years ago by Don Kendall, PepsiCo's former chairman and chief executive officer. He still holds to this philosophy in his position as chairman of the executive committee of PepsiCo's board of directors. And his views on physical fitness are shared by his successor, Wayne Calloway, and by many others throughout PepsiCo.

We at PepsiCo believe that health and physical fitness programs make a significant contribution to the well-being of our employees and, consequently, to our business. Physical fitness programs have been a part of PepsiCo for more than a quarter of a century. In the early 1960s PepsiCo headquarters were in New York City. Even though space was at a premium, an executive fitness center was part of the corporate headquarters.

At the time the center was open only to senior management. In 1970, when we moved our headquarters to Purchase, New York, we expanded the fitness center and opened it to middle management as well. By the end of the 1970s we decided to expand our health and fitness programs once again and to make them available to all the employees working in our corporate headquarters.

PepsiCo opened a new fitness center for the 700 people at our corporate headquarters in 1981. It occupies over 12,000 square feet and provides a full range of exercise equipment, programs, and professional supervision. The center immediately proved very popular with our employees, who used it before and after work and during available break time.

The success at our corporate fitness center encouraged us to establish similar fitness and related health education programs in each of our divisions (Pepsi-Cola headquarters in Somers and Valhalla, New York; Frito-Lay's headquarters in Plano, Texas; PepsiCo Foods International headquarters in Dallas; Taco Bell in Irvine, California; and Pizza Hut in

169

Wichita). All operate modern fitness centers with extensive programs available to all employees. In addition, Kentucky Fried Chicken, a company we acquired in 1986, is studying the feasibility of constructing a new fitness center for its headquarters' employees in Louisville, Kentucky.

We regard the money we spend to build and maintain these fitness centers as an investment in our employees. Our employees tell us that they feel our on-site fitness programs show that we care about their well-being. The fitness facility says something about the lifestyle and philosophy of the company that the employees share and appreciate.

The fitness center also has proved to be a very effective recruiting tool. Prospective employees see the facilities and the programs we offer as an added benefit of employment. That means we attract the kind of people who have healthy, fit, and productive lifestyles. Independent research studies have demonstrated that healthy and fit people are more productive and have lower rates of absenteeism than those who are not. We accept the validity of these studies and have used them as the scientific basis for our employee programs.

Our headquarters' work force is large enough to make it cost-effective to build and staff fitness center facilities. The workers have primarily white-collar, sedentary jobs, and most understand the importance of health and fitness. They are also the driving force within the corporate culture. They provide an example that others tend to follow.

Delivering the same kind of cost-effective programs to our blue collar workers at plant sites and in our restaurant business presents us with different problems. We have almost a quarter of a million employees scattered all over the country, indeed, the world. It is far more difficult to deliver fitness programs to these people than to our corporate employees.

Plant and restaurant employees, for instance, have fixed working schedules. The production line cannot be stopped when a worker decides to exercise. The number of employees at our plant sites, moreover, is significantly smaller than at our headquarters. Building costs alone seem to prevent construction of fitness centers at each of these plant sites. To investigate some of these problems, the PepsiCo Foundation, established in 1982 to coordinate the company's charitable contributions, funded a major research study to determine how to provide a cost-effective, low-level health intervention program for our plant employees.

The project, known as "Lifeline," studied employees at two of our larger Frito-Lay plants (at Charlotte, North Carolina, and Killingly, Connecticut); they served as an experimental group. Frito-Lay employees at plants in Frankford, Indiana, and Topeka, Kansas, served as a matched control group.

The employees at these four plants underwent health and fitness evaluations at the start and end of the 1-year experiment. As part of the project we developed specific health education material, provided health counseling, and offered other direct services to promote better health and fitness.

We have not completed our analysis of the physical data from this study, but we have learned some very practical things from the project. The employees' attitude toward the company has improved significantly. They came to see the project as evidence that the company cared about them. They felt, in effect, that the company was saying, "We care about your health and fitness. Even more important, we care about you."

We also learned that health counselors could play an important role in employee relations. We chose these counselors both for their technical skills and because they could relate well to the plant workers. The plant employees did not view the health counselors as part of management, and this put them in a very special position. The plant workers quickly developed a trust in the health counselors, which made it possible for them not only to influence health behavior but also to help both management and labor with job-related problems. The workers received the benefits of health education and advice from counselors they respected, and management also received the advice of the health counselors on job-related problems.

Another thing we learned from the PepsiCo Foundation–sponsored study was that the involvement of the employees at a grass-roots level was important to the success of the program. The employees felt it was "their" program. Whether the employees were involved with the counselors or working on their own, the program was well received by most. When management added its support, we had all the right factors in place for success. Last year we completed the formal part of the funded research at the two experimental and the two control plants. We are now expanding beyond these four sites to all 37 of our Frito-Lay plants.

The cost involved and the benefits received are a legitimate concern of any program we have. Thus far in the physical fitness program we have seen benefits that are hard to quantify. We cannot yet say that for every dollar we spend we are getting a positive return on the investment. Because we cannot quantify the hard dollar savings our health and fitness programs provide, we believe it is important to keep the dollar cost down and administrative overhead low. This year we are trying to expand our low-cost health intervention program in all our Frito-Lay plants. We are using the original four-plant health counselors as regional health advisors to our other plant locations.

These health counselors are responsible for generating initial interest. We think it is important for employees at each plant to develop ownership for the programs by forming employee health committees and gaining the support of the plant managers. When this is done, the designated area health counselor can help them in organizing and developing the program. This approach is in its infancy, so it is too early to report on its progress.

Our Pepsi-Cola plant employees are typical of production workers at Frito-Lay, but the route sales people at both companies have special job duties that can lead to major health problems. They are responsible for moving and delivering some very heavy containers. During a normal day's service, any one of our 17,000 route sales people can move as much as 7 tons of our product. We are trying to turn the special job requirements of a route salesworker into a means of motivating drivers to become interested in health and to take better care of themselves. We are conducting a pilot project in Orlando, Florida, to determine the health value of having these sales people participate in physical conditioning programs.

The presumption of this pilot program is that those who are physically fit should experience fewer sprains and strains. One problem we find is convincing the sales force of the value of regular fitness training. Those who move tons of weight a day tend to feel that they do not need any additional exercise. Despite this one problem, we have found the sales people do have genuine interest in fitness and the other areas of health promotion we offer, specifically in weight management and nutrition.

Our three restaurant divisions—Pizza Hut, Taco Bell, and Kentucky Fried Chicken—present us with an even more challenging problem in promoting cost-effective fitness and health because 95% of these employees are in small local units. The issue is, How do we convince these almost 100,000 employees that health and fitness are important to their well-being and do this in a cost-effective manner? We have not yet answered that question.

PepsiCo is a people-intensive company. We are the ninth largest employer in the United States and have 225,000 employees worldwide. These people are our biggest asset, and we must protect them as we would any important investment. This attitude explains why PepsiCo is a leader in employee health and fitness programs. All our employees are important to us. Providing health and fitness programs is one way of demonstrating that. We also want to send another message to our employees—that a lifestyle of staying fit and keeping healthy is important for our employees. Such a lifestyle helps our employees have healthier, happier, and more productive personal lives and helps them perform to their fullest potential while on the job.

Our goal is to develop programs that will reach everyone. We want to do more than provide programs that attract only those who are already fit. We want to concentrate on the group of employees who are sedentary and have other health risks, such as overweight, hypertension, high cholesterol, or smoking. We need to educate our employees that healthy and fit lifestyles are beneficial not only to the company but also to them. The major thrust of our future program development will pivot around a series of questions: How do we make health programs a part of the workplace? How do we make these programs cost effective? How do we motivate those who have little interest in changing unhealthy lifestyles?

The list of questions can go on. They all come down to one deceptively simple question: How do we reach the 95% of our employees we are not reaching now? This question has to be answered by all employers. When we answer it, we can reach our goal of delivering health and fitness programs to all our employees. This is our goal—because "you can't run a successful company with people only 'half well.' "

Corporate Health Promotion—Today and Tomorrow

Frank H. Barker

Johnson & Johnson Health Management, Inc.,
New Brunswick, New Jersey

It is a pleasure to be able to discuss corporate health promotion as we at Johnson & Johnson assess it today and as we see tomorrow's developments. The "today" segment reflects our experience with health promotion within our company and also with other employers as we embark on our new health promotion commercial venture—the Johnson & Johnson Health Management company.

In the mid-1970s we became aware of the increasing public interest in health, reflected in many ways but perhaps most noticeably in the growing amount of TV programming devoted to health topics. Health-oriented TV programming has grown from approximately 100 hours in 1974 to 2,578 hours in 1987. The networks and independents would not have increased their programming so dramatically without viewer interest as measured by audience ratings. During this same period employee health care costs rose at unacceptable rates as the public interest in health was increasing.

We concluded in the late 1970s that a properly designed, medically and scientifically based, measurable health promotion program would be well received by our managements and employees and possibly would offer significant health benefits to our human capital as well as economic and employee commitment benefits to the company. We felt our employees were eager to take greater responsibility for their health.

With the help of outside experts, such as Paul Stolley of the University of Pennsylvania, Bob Shipley of Duke, Lester Breslow of UCLA, Johanna Dwyer of Tufts, and others, we developed a health promotion system to meet our objectives. The Live for Life® system was tested epidemiologically and attitudinally from 1980 to 1982 with approximately 3,500 Johnson & Johnson employees—2,000 in test companies and 1,500 in control companies. We recognize that 2 years is a limited time frame for a longitudinal epidemiological study, but it served as an important beginning. Additionally, we had the Research Triangle Institute measure employee reaction to the Live for Life® program.

173

We asked Wharton School economists to study from 1979 to 1983 the impact of our Live for Life® system on the health care costs of 5,000 employees, compared with 3,000 employees in Johnson & Johnson companies without a health promotion program. Efforts were made to choose control sites where employee populations closely resembled those of the study group. The system comprises five components:

1. Health assessment
2. Promotional support
3. Health improvement programs
4. Site management
5. Management information system

All components are important—from the 1-hr nurse-administered health assessment; to the core programmatic component emphasizing smoking cessation, exercise, weight management, cholesterol control, nutrition, stress management, and blood pressure control; to the on-site manager using effective and frequently refreshed promotional materials to generate participation; to the management information system to measure results compared with objectives.

It is important to keep in mind that the measurements made at Johnson & Johnson were based on the total employee population, not just those who participated. This is a key point because senior managements are interested in the impact of the system on all of their employees, not just on active program participants. All employees, both blue and white collar, are eligible at each Johnson & Johnson work site.

At each site we had an average of 90% participation in the initial health assessment, and annually we average approximately 60% employee participation in one or more lifestyle change or health improvement programs. The participation level is by far the most important element because it is the major determinant of program success. When you obtain majority participation, you will have a positive impact on employee health and attitudes and health care costs. Majority participation achieves a cultural change at the work site, which gives permanency to health promotion. We believe it takes a coordinated and integrated systems approach to change the work site culture to one of positive health orientation.

The degree of participation by blue-collar and white-collar employees is similar; there is no statistically significant difference. Later I will mention some of the barriers we dealt with in achieving similar levels of participation. The following are some of our study results.

We tripled the 2-year natural smoking quit rate (23% vs. 8%) in the employee test population with the full Live for Life® system. This measurement is against all smokers and is a long-term (14-month) quit rate verified by thiocyanate. Control companies (represented by health profiles) indicate the assessment is an intervention tool with modest success. Of the smokers who attended the smoking cessation program, 40% quit.

The test group of employees as a whole reduced both systolic and diastolic blood pressure over the 2 years, while the control group reflected a normative increase with age. All of these changes were statistically significant and especially impressive when viewed from a public health viewpoint of large employee populations.

Using maximum oxygen uptake as a measurement of cardiovascular fitness, the Live for Life® employees reached slightly more than 50% of the maximum change attainable. The important finding here was the broad-based nature of the group whose fitness was improved. We were successful in getting a similar percentage from each cardiovascular risk quartile, including the higher risk, sedentary lifestyle employees, to exercise. The result was not caused by a select group of 10K runners becoming marathoners. We were pleased that the *Journal of The American Medical Association* accepted Steve Blair's study of this program for publication in its February 1986 issue.

From both employee-health and economic viewpoints, we were delighted with the decrease of absenteeism among test employees. The 15% reduction occurred primarily within the production and clerical employee populations. It is interesting to note that the control group experienced an increase in absenteeism.

An impressive economic gain was demonstrated in employee hospital costs between the 5,000 Live for Life® employees and the 3,000 employees without our health promotion system. We were successful in slowing the rate of increase in hospital costs for Live for Life® employees compared with the control group. The year 1979 was the base measurement period for both groups. Johnson & Johnson employees in the Live for Life® group began participating during 1980 and the first half of 1981. By the end of 1982 a 17% difference in hospital costs existed between the two groups—and by 1983 the difference was 34%. Wharton economists performed the study, adjusting for all variables except Live for Life®. The study was published in the *Journal of The American Medical Association* in December 1986.

As previously mentioned, we had the Research Triangle Institute monitor employee satisfaction in the test and control companies. Statistically significant differences were noted in these areas:

- Satisfaction with supervision
- Commitment to the organization
- Satisfaction with working conditions
- Satisfaction with pay and fringe benefits
- Sense of job security

The Johnson & Johnson family of companies has minimal variations in personnel policies, compensation and benefits, and working conditions. Therefore, we attributed these employee relations benefits to the Live for Life® system in the test population. The increase in the sense of job security was particularly gratifying.

We were and are pleased with these and other results, especially since we have expanded to more than 75 Johnson & Johnson locations with approximately 33,000 employees as well as to other corporations.

In summary, we define the Live for Life® Health Promotion System as follows: Live for Life® is a proven, adaptable work site health promotion system that motivates a majority of employees to make long-term improvements in their health habits. The system measurably reduces health care and other operating costs and improves employee company commitment. The key definition components are that the system is proven, adaptable, measured, and motivates a majority of employees.

It was not easy to attain the objectives we set for the program, and there were many barriers. The most significant was that management generally was skeptical of the returns on investment in workplace health promotion. However, our test results—primarily economic returns and employee health and relations gains—convinced most of our company managements to implement Live for Life®. (Nothing breeds success like success.) As we expanded, word that the program was worthwhile passed among Johnson & Johnson companies. Although management participation initially was spotty, it has grown commensurate with managers' realization of the benefits.

There were also several employee barriers. First was gaining access to ensure thorough communication at all levels. We convinced management to provide company time for all employees, hourly and salaried, to attend orientation sessions and to participate in the initial health assessment. Also, we suggested and had approved a policy regarding the ongoing health improvement programs. The programs would be provided free to all employees, but employees would participate on their time. In setting this policy, the concept of partnership was effected.

A continual employee barrier is loss of interest. As with any effective marketing program, we periodically refresh the promotional support package that surrounds our core health improvement programs to maintain high awareness and participation. Special events, multimedia programming, increased family communication, new and refined programs—all contribute to the maintenance of employee interest and participation.

One note about blue-collar workers: As previously mentioned, we have equivalent participation by blue-collar employees. To achieve this, it is necessary (a) to be flexible in programming the system to meet the needs of shift workers, (b) to take extra time to communicate to all production employees and, if represented, to their union managements, and (c) not to segregate facilities, education classes, or special events by blue- or white-collar employee status.

Maintaining consistent quality at all locations was an initial barrier to success and always is a major concern. Locating, attracting, and training administrators and program leaders also is a challenge, but there can be no compromise in this area. Programs must be implemented to specifications by qualified and certified personnel. We found it necessary to initiate and maintain a training school for our administrators and program leaders.

Determining appropriate data and a data collection system was another barrier. With assistance from outside experts and our management information center, we developed an information system for employees and managements that enables ongoing measurement and reporting of results versus objectives for each work site.

That's today. Now let's look forward and identify some trends and forecasts. Planning will take a quantum leap. More sophisticated techniques will be used to assess individual workplace needs, wants, and capabilities. Health promotion implementation will be studied and planned as extensively as environmental safety, employee productivity, machine efficiency, employee benefits redesign, and other areas vitally important to the success of industry. At Johnson & Johnson Health Management, we conduct this study via tactical planning at each workplace, usually over 60 to 90 days.

We believe employers will increasingly accept health promotion. It is the longer term solution—perhaps the only solution—to health care costs, and it improves employee commitment and productivity. Employers will have to invest adequately to achieve their economic and employee relations objectives. Smaller employers will embrace health promotion to a greater degree as proven delivery systems evolve for their employee populations. More managements will conclude that managing health is as good an objective or a better one than trying to manage the health care that employees and dependents receive.

Employee acceptance will increase also. More comprehensive and proven programs, properly marketed, will gain increased employee participation. As this occurs, expanded programs will be well received by positive health-oriented employee populations. More restrictive smoking policies, drug and alcohol education and testing, and AIDS education will be more easily understood and supported by employees who sense their employers are truly interested in their well-being.

Programs that interrelate multiple health improvement activities will be most successful in effecting long-term change. With smoking, for example, programs that incorporate exercise, stress management, and weight management in addition to smoking cessation are more likely to have greater appeal and better results. Improved delivery methods and increased investment in health promotion programs for dependents and retirees will occur. Family and retiree involvement will add to the epidemiological and economic gains, and these will be documented.

On-site delivery, especially for larger workplaces, will increase because the evidence is becoming more clear that majority participation occurs when the convenience factor is high. Participation leads to results. Greater control of the program, better integration of program elements, and better recognition of the employer's concern for employees—all result from on-site delivery. Community resource-based delivery also will increase as "hard-to-reach" employee populations (e.g., sales and service representatives, small groups), dependents, and retirees are offered health promotion.

Research and development will increase significantly. The science is evolving. Delivery and teaching methodologies are improving. Some targets of this research and development are likely to be these:

- Effective health promotion programs for older employees and retirees
- Family-oriented health promotion programs
- Program development for "hard-core," extremely difficult-to-change employees and a more personalized approach
- Better longitudinal tracking of individual participant progress
- Utilization of health promotion risk data in underwriting health and life insurance

We are very pleased to be working with the Duke University Medical Center in research and development. The creation of a health promotion clinical laboratory at Duke via linkage of the DUPAC Program with their cardiovascular data base will provide an excellent testing facility.

I have emphasized the need for proven programs many times. The demand for proof is great today. It is required to gain increased acceptance. We believe proven programs will move the health promotion industry forward more rapidly.

Corporate health promotion is a reality today, but the opportunity for tomorrow is enormous. There are huge benefits for everyone. It is a triple-win situation for employer, employees, and suppliers. I encourage all of us to work diligently and professionally to expand this very important movement and to create a soundly based, professional industry.

The majority of the work force that will start the next century is at work today. Therefore, it is not only advantageous but vital to improve our competitive positions. A healthier work force is more productive and committed. We have a long way to go, but the journey is exciting and rewarding.

Conference Participants

Frank H. Barker, President
Johnson & Johnson Health
  Management, Inc.
501 George Street
Kilmer House K-502
New Brunswick, NJ 08903

Edward J. Bernacki
Vice President for Medical Affairs
Tenneco Incorporated
P.O. Box 2511, Suite 1047
Houston, TX 77252

Perry J. Blackshear
Division of Endocrinology
Box 3897
Duke University Medical Center
Durham, NC 27710

Frank W. Booth
Department of Physiology and
  Cell Biology
The University of Texas
Medical School
P.O. Box 20708
Houston, TX 77225

Harvey J. Cohen
Division of Geriatrics
Box 3003
Duke University Medical Center
Durham, NC 27710

Fredrick L. Dunn
Division of Endocrinology
Box 3939
Duke University Medical Center
Durham, NC 27710

Irwin Fridovich
Department of Biochemistry
Box 3711
Duke University Medical Center
Durham, NC 27710

William L. Haskell
Stanford University
School of Medicine
730 Welch Road, Suite B
Palo Alto, CA 94304

Barton F. Haynes
Division of Rheumatology and
  Immunology
Box 3258
Duke University Medical Center
Durham, NC 27710

J. Roger King
Personnel Director
PepsiCo, Inc.
Anderson Hill Road
Purchase, NY 10577

Jere H. Mitchell
Department of Internal Medicine
The Pauline and Adolph
  Weinberger Lab for Cardiology
  Research
University of Texas, Health
  Science Center
5323 Harry Hines Boulevard
Dallas, TX 75235

Max L. Morton, Manager
Wellness Services
Adolph Coors Company
Golden, CO 80401

Lester Packer
Department of Physiology–
    Anatomy
University of California at
    Berkeley
Berkeley, CA 94720

Erik A. Richter
August Krogh Institute
University of Copenhagen
Universitetsparken 13
DK-2100 Copenhagen O
Denmark

Judith Rodin
Department of Psychology
Yale University
P.O. Box 11A, Yale Station
New Haven, CT 06520

Bengt Saltin
August Krogh Institute
University of Copenhagen
Universitetsparken 13
DK-2100 Copenhagen O
Denmark

Roy J. Shephard
Department of Preventive
    Medicine and Biostatistics
University of Toronto
Toronto, Ontario
Canada M5S 1A1

Andrew G. Wallace
Department of Medicine
Box 3708
Duke University Medical Center
Durham, NC 27710

Jay M. Weiss, Professor
Department of Psychiatry
Box 3829
Duke University Medical Center
Durham, NC 27710

R. Sanders Williams
Department of Medicine
Box 3945
Duke University Medical Center
Durham, NC 27710

Peter D. Wood
Professor of Medicine
Stanford University
Stanford, CA 94305